WAISTLINE WORKSHOP

CHARTWELL
BOOKS INC.

Editor Brenda Marshall
Designer Monica Jones
Cover design David Robinson

© Marshall Cavendish Limited 1978
All rights reserved

This book is not to be sold outside the United States
of America, its territories and Canada

Printed in the United Kingdom

Published by Chartwell Books Inc.
A Division of Book Sales Inc.
110 Enterprise Avenue
Secaucus, New Jersey 07094

ISBN 0 89009 168 4

NB American terminology is indicated in the text by
( ) brackets

Pictures supplied by:
Robyn Beeche 65 and front cover; Alan Duns 36-37, 47;
Paul Kemp 18, 34; Nigel Messett 16, 17; Kim Sayer 44;
M. Scoular 39; Syndication International 13, 15

Pictures researched by Jackum Brown, Alice Peebles

All other photography by Naru

Material used in the Nutrition Chart and in the table
on Energy consumed in some common activities, is based
on statistics in The Manual of Nutrition, eighth edition,
and in The Composition of Foods (R.A. McCance and
E.M. Widdowson), and is quoted by kind permission of
Her Majesty's Stationery Office

The height and weight charts are based on those drawn up
by the Metropolitan Life Insurance Company, New York

INTRODUCTION

Nothing looks better, or feels better for that matter, than a trim, healthy body that is carrying no excess fat — and this should be the goal of men and women alike.

Discover why you eat too much and why it's important to eat a balanced diet, even when you're slimming. **Waistline Workshop** will show you that you don't need to starve yourself to get slim: re-educate your eating habits so that once you've reached your ideal weight you can remain there.

Slimming can be fun using **Waistline Workshop's** authoritative, yet easy to use, nutrition chart to plan your meals. You can choose the foods you really like and maybe try some new ones you didn't realize were so nutritious yet low in Calories. In fact, counting Calories should not be looked upon as a chore — you might think it a waste of time, but remember, while you're counting Calories you're not nibbling titbits through boredom.

Sensible eating is the major part of staying slim but healthy exercise is also important and **Waistline Workshop** has selected special exercise to tone and firm specific parts of the body — so you can use them as a general keep fit routine or simply do those designed for your 'problem' areas.

Let **Waistline Workshop** show you the way to a new and slimmer you the healthy way.

CONTENTS

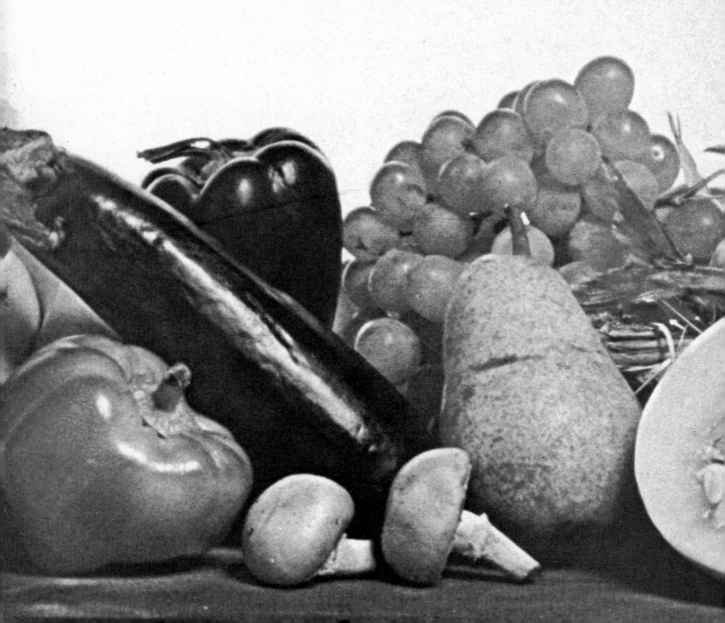

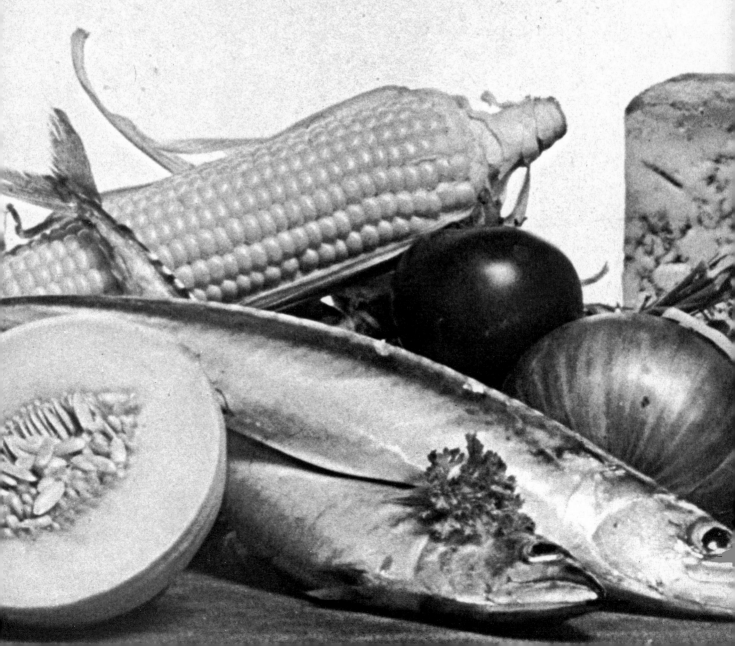

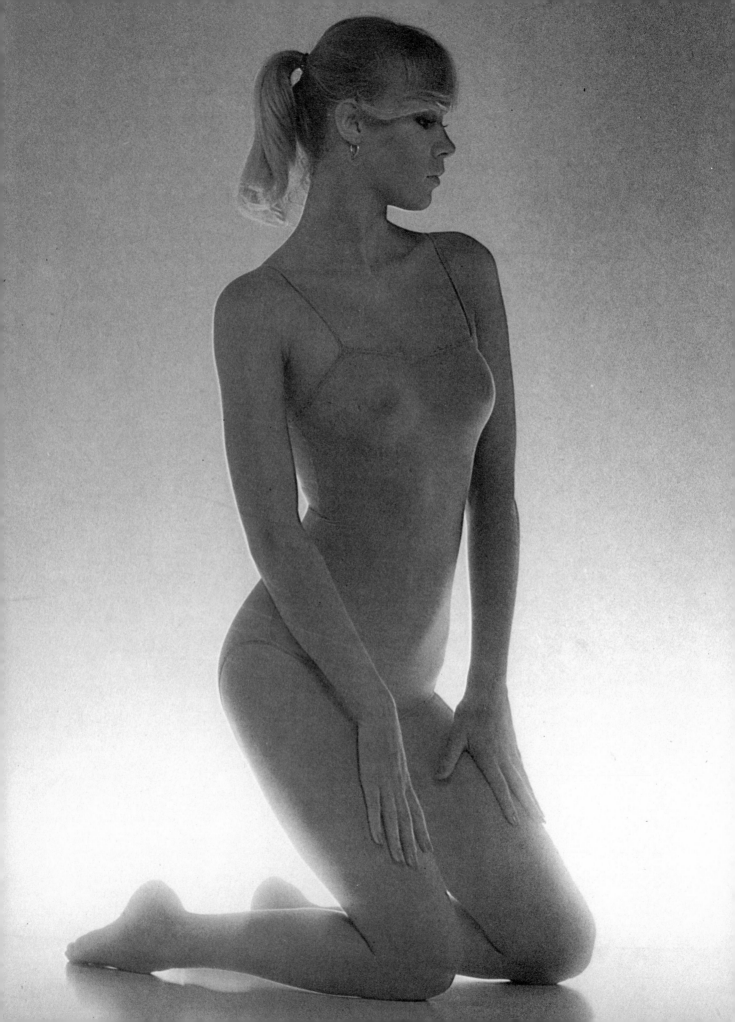

SHAPING UP
THE PERFECT SHAPE?

The search for the perfect shape has been going on for centuries but what *is* the perfect shape? Does the perfect shape for the male or female body exist or is it an ideal, attainable only by a Pygmalion able to mould a body to a perfect figure and then bring it to life?

Doctors are not particularly interested in body shape except in so far as disease and shape are sometimes connected, so it is to the artists and fahion trendsetters that we turn to ask if an ideal does exist. In fact, fashions change so rapidly nowadays that you may go through three or four different shapes in your lifespan.

Once the classic proportion for a female body was that the distance from the breast to the navel should be the same as the distance from the navel to the top of the legs. Yet in the Middle Ages, the Gothic centuries, the ideal female form showed an elongated oval-shaped body, with the distance from the breast to the navel almost twice that of the navel to the top of the legs. Think of the unisex fashion of today, the boyish Twiggy era and, even earlier, the broad-shouldered military look of the forties. Whatever body shape fashion dictated, the beauty conscious woman would strive to attain it.

Who does the ideal male body exist for? Perhaps only for other men who feel they are themselves unattractive to women. Certainly it seems that the perfect male shape as portrayed in Michelangelo's David is far from being generally admired by women. Men imagine that women admire muscles, big shoulders and huge biceps. Yet current opinion polls show that what turns most women on about a man's body are small, sexy buttocks and a slim, flat stomach, though women do not normally assess men by physique alone.

So art and fashion tell us that the perfect shape, the ideal of beauty, lies only in the eye of the beholder, an eye that sees largely what the most admired men and women of the age look like and then strives to be like them. Can science, and more especially medicine, help? Medicine puts forward as the ideal shape 'the body that is most satisfactorily adjusted to its environment'. Not a glamorous ideal at first, but if you examine the facts, it is the only sensible one.

This fact is even more apparent when we think of the many different races and cultures throughout the world. Each different race has its own ideals of beauty and perfection. What appeals to an Eskimo as beautiful and attractive would probably not appeal to the European. Take the giraffe-necked women of the Padaung tribe: their elongated necks are considered beautiful by their men, yet to the European mind it would appear to be a distortion of beauty.

You must be practical and realize that while you can alter your shape to a certain degree to suit current trends and fashions, you cannot alter your basic framework. Although physique varies from person to person your basic bone structure is decided at birth and is with you for your entire life. The best way of identifying your body type is through 'somatotyping'. This is a method of body classification developed in the 1940s by American psychologist W. H. Sheldon. He carried out studies on thousands of Americans and found that everyone could be categorized into just three basic bodily shapes or somatotypes—endomorph, mesomorph and ectomorph.

The endomorph is essentially rounded with relatively short limbs and quite often a protruding stomach which adds to the roundness. Their hips are often wider than their shoulders. Although endomorphs are generally heavily built and more inclined to put on weight, they need not necessarily be fat. As people in this group are fairly relaxed and not too energetic in movement, the wise endomorphs should pay extra attention to their diet, avoiding even a few pounds of excess weight.

The muscular mesomorph has the figure of the classic Grecian athlete—wide shoulders, broad chest, narrow hips and muscular arms and legs. This group is generally more physically active than the others, so is less likely to carry any excess fat. Women are less common in this group as the more muscular tendencies in men are related to the male sex hormone testosterone, produced by the testes.

The ectomorph has a thin, narrow angular body. Shoulders and hips are narrow with very little evidence of fat or muscle. Very few ectomorphs become overweight and it is thought that they have the best health of the three groups.

Everyone is a mixture of these three groups although belonging primarily to one. The simplest way to recognize your own body type is to stand in front of a mirror naked, and ask yourself if your body has the appearance of the wide and rounded endomorph, the long narrowness of the ectomorph or the muscular broad chest and narrow hips of the mesomorph.

Once you have discovered your own body type you must accept that it has certain limitations within its own framework. For instance, no amount of dieting will make the rounded figure of the endomorph become a thin ectomorph. It will still remain rounded though without any excess flesh.

It is in everyone's power to make the best of himself or herself. You can control what you look like. And the way to do this is to see that the way you live, your adjustment to your environment, are right for you.

Your perfect shape is that at which you are happiest.

BODY IMAGE

Whether you are an endomorph, ectomorph or mesomorph your overall body image will depend greatly on how you feel and carry yourself. Knowing you look your best will give you an inner confidence which really does reflect in your total appearance. A trim, healthy body, full of vigour and vitality, should be your constant goal.

First you need to recognize your faults. Take a long, critical look at yourself in a full length mirror. Are you happy with what you see? Can you make any improvements? Wide hips that are due to bone structure you can do nothing about, but wide hips due to excess fat you can. Try to distinguish between characteristics caused by bone structure and faults caused by you. After all, you are the one responsible for your overall appearance: you choose the food you eat and the life you lead. Your general way of life and diet reflect in the condition of your body, hair, nails and especially skin and eyes.

Often a great deal of what appears to be too much flesh is due not to overeating, but to bad posture. A simple test to see if your 'tummy' is due to too much food or bad posture is to lie flat on your back. If your tummy disappears, it is your posture that needs attention rather than your eating habits. A tummy from too much food would not disappear.

Improving your carriage and posture will do a great deal to improve your shape and appearance. It will probably be the answer to many aches and pains as well.

Good posture will also give your internal organs a chance to do their work properly. Sagging shoulders are one of the worst offenders of bad posture and all too often a habit carried over from childhood. When the shoulders sag forward, the chest becomes cramped and the lungs are unable to expand fully. This, of course, limits the amount of oxygen breathed in, which can often result in tiredness and lack of energy. If food cannot be properly processed after a meal, because the stomach and intestines have been regularly cramped from not sitting straight while eating, faulty digestive and bowel function may follow.

Sitting and walking with your head held forward puts unnecessary strain on the muscles at the back of the neck and upper back causing backache. Good posture strengthens muscles and ligaments enabling you to move more energetically and gracefully.

So, by simply improving your posture you will not only look better and move with more grace, you will actually feel better because your entire body will be functioning correctly.

Here are a few simple posture points to bear in mind.

Sitting
Wherever possible choose a hard chair to sit in, especially if you are to be seated for long periods. As well as being better for the buttock muscles, you will find it more comfortable. If you are sitting down to work at a desk or table make sure that the chair and working surface are the correct height. Your knees should fit comfortably under the table and the surface should be easily accessible without any unnecessary bending at the waist.

Sitting down and rising from a chair should be done as one flowing movement. When sitting, lower yourself gently into a chair, placing your bottom into the back of the seat so that your hip joint forms a right angle. Press your thighs evenly over the seat of the chair and keep your stomach and buttock muscles taut. Keep your knees together, feet flat on the floor and hold your legs straight or with knees bent slightly to left or right. Try not to cross your legs when sitting down as this does tend to impede the flow of blood. Hold your back straight, with shoulders back and relaxed. Don't let them slouch forward or you will end up with backache. Once you get used to sitting correctly you will find it much more comfortable to sit for longer periods.

Standing
Always stand straight and tall with your spine stretched fully and head held back. Your chin should be parallel to the ground. Keep your tummy muscles pulled in and contract buttock muscles so that the seat is well tucked under. Keep your shoulders pulled back and down but completely relaxed, and let your arms hang loosely by your sides. Make sure that your weight is balanced evenly on both feet and hips kept level. Never tilt your hips to one side so that all your weight is on one leg. If your standing posture is correct, a straight line drawn from just behind your ear would pass vertically through your shoulders, arms, legs and ankles.

Walking
Walking should be an enjoyable and totally relaxed movement. Hold your back straight, head up and shoulders back. Walk tall and proud swinging each leg from the hip—not from the knees. Tilt your body slightly forward as your weight transfers from the back to the front foot. Let the movement be natural and easy with arms swinging gently at your sides. Try to keep your breathing regular as you walk. A rhythm of breathing slowly and deeply to a count of four in, four out is a good habit to get into.

Bending
Bending down to lift heavy objects is often another unnecessary strain, generally put on the back. It is the legs, arms and stomach muscles that should be taking the strain. Lower yourself by bending at the knees. Let your arms take the weight of the object and use your legs and stomach muscles to straighten up again. You only need to try it once to see that it makes sense.

Short, tall or medium—make the most of your body image.

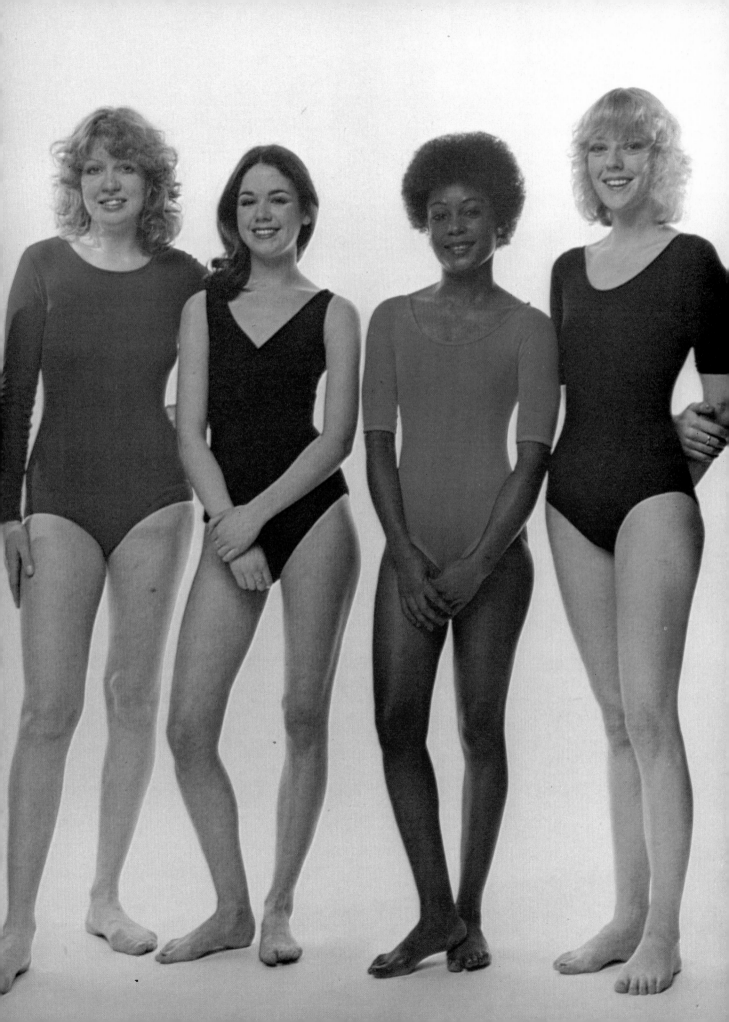

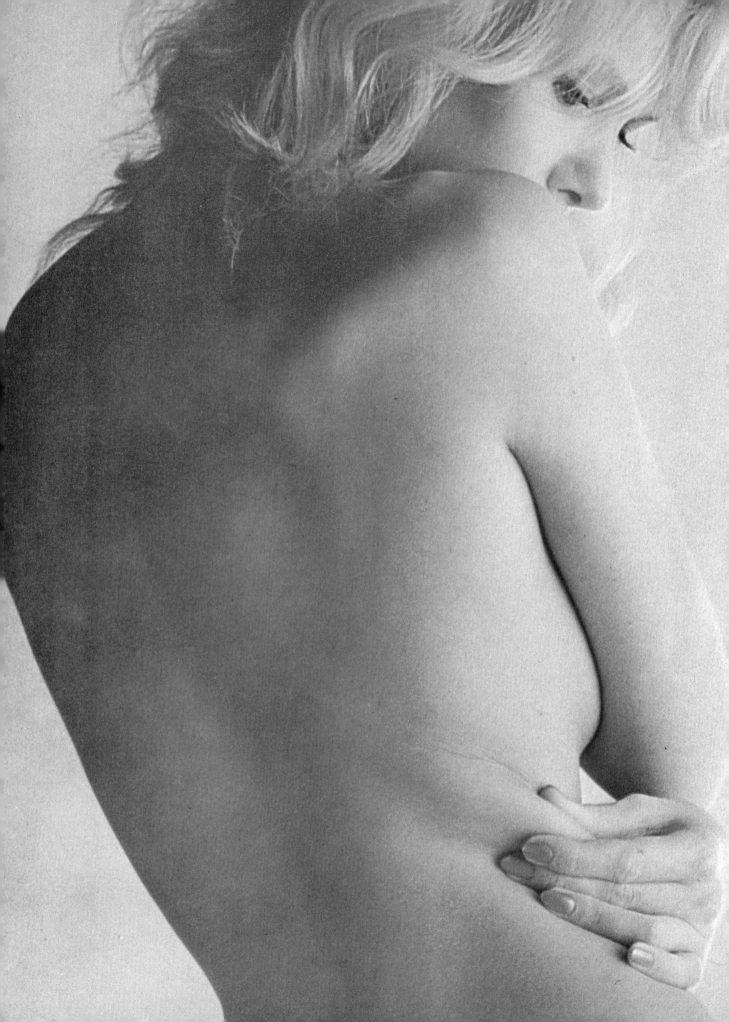

MEASURE UP

Are you overweight? Is it time to start a reducing diet? If there is any part of your body, thighs, bottom, stomach, that you feel could be improved, then the answer is probably yes. Measuring excess fat is not easy but a simple way to test if your extra weight is just fat is to try the 'pinch' test. Take skin between your thumb and first finger from any of the fat prone areas—just below the shoulder blade, the back of the upper arm, the midriff and inner thighs. If you can pinch more than an inch of skin you can consider yourself overweight and ready to shed that excess fat.

Because people do vary so much in shape and build, no one weight can be right for everyone of the same height and sex. Someone who is carrying extra weight need not be fat; the extra weight could be firm muscle. Your ideal weight is really that at which you feel your best. A height and weight table can give you a rough idea of what you should weigh for your particular frame, but you must remember that it is only a guide. For instance if you look at the heaviest desirable weight for a man standing 1.9m [6ft 4in] it is 92.5 kilos [204 pounds]. Does that mean, therefore, that a Mr Universe weighing around 107.9 kilos [238 pounds] is overweight? No, nor could you find any excess fat on him or many other athletes in the same position—the additional weight comes from well developed muscles. On the other hand, a man with a 'paunch' may not be overweight, although he may look fat. What he needs is exercise to redistribute the excess flesh and to restore the tone of the muscles that have allowed his belly to sag.

There is another problem when keeping a check on your weight and that is that it does tend to vary from day to day, especially in women during the days before menstruation. A woman may add about a kilo or more [two to three pounds] to her weight, and, very occasionally some women have been known to put on an extra four and a half kilos [10 pounds]. This gain in weight is due to water retention, particularly in the breasts and abdominal area, rather than fat accumulation—and it is only temporary.

This accumulation of fluid is due to the increased level of the hormone oestrogen (or estrogen), which influences the salt/water balance in the body, reducing the amount of salt and water that is excreted by the kidneys. But as menstruation starts the estrogen level drops, salt and water retention decreases, more urine is passed and weight returns to normal.

Another probable cause of fluid retention can be the Pill. Some women notice a gain of up to three and a half kilos [seven pounds] during the first three to four months on the contraceptive Pill, although much higher figures have been recorded. However, fluid retention is only true of some cases: the extra weight could be due to overeating. Increased contentment from being on the Pill may make a woman eat more, or the exact opposite, depression (which can also be a side effect of the Pill) may be the cause of overeating. The menopause is also marked by weight changes caused by fluid retention and hormonal balance.

So the wise slimmer who wants to keep track of her progress will not only keep track of weight, but also measurements. Keeping a written record of your weight and measurements during the first weeks of dieting can be a good incentive to carry on with your reducing diet. It is during the first few weeks that weight will be lost fairly quickly because by eating less carbohydrates, the body's own sugar stores are called upon for energy, resulting in a loss of fluid. But after this initial loss a 'block' seems to occur and it is at this time that you need the extra incentive and determination to carry on. The rate at which you continue to lose the extra pounds will depend on the diet you choose.

No one can tell you how much you will lose in a week, a month or a year simply because no two people are alike. You can put five men or women on exactly the same diet and at the end of three months they might have lost, say, five and a half kilos [12 pounds] each. But it is improbable that they would all have lost an equal amount when they had been on the diet for only six weeks. This is because the loss of water and its effect on the balance of water remaining in the body varies in each one of us and each body will take its own time to return to a normal water balance.

However, a rough guide for weight loss would be about three kilos [seven pounds] in one month, six and a half kilos [14 pounds] up to three months, and a sensible weekly loss would be 900 grams to 1.3 kilos [two to three pounds] until your ideal weight is reached. Then remain on a sensibly balanced diet with calorie intake matching energy output. As soon as you go a half to one kilo [one to two pounds] over, cut down on the calories immediately.

Weigh in
Always weigh yourself at the same time of the day—not every day because of weight fluctuation—preferably with bladder and bowels empty.
Try to wear the same clothes each time you weigh yourself, otherwise weigh in the nude.
Use the same scales and make sure they are on an even floor, not sinking into a thick carpet.
Stand on the centre of the machine with your weight evenly distributed on heels and balls of the feet.

Measure up
Use a substantial tape that hasn't stretched with wear.
Measure around breast or chest, waist and hips.
Place the tape in exactly the same place each time or the results will be inaccurate.

Always keep a regular check on your body to avoid fat build-up in any area. If you can pinch too thick a fold of skin between your fingers, it's time to cut down on the carbohydrates and try a little exercise.

HIGH IDEALS

A simple way to gauge your frame
If you are a woman measure your wrist.
If it measures 13.5 cm [5½ in] or less, you have a small frame; between 13.5 cm and 16 cm [5½ and 6¼ in] is a medium frame; 16 cm [6¼ in] and over is a large frame.
If you are a man measure chest, width of shoulders and length of hands and feet.
Chest 96 cm [38 in], shoulders 42.5 cm [17 in], hand 17.5 cm [7 in], foot 20 cm [8 in] or less would be a small frame;
Chest 112 cm [44 in], shoulders 52.5 cm [21 in], hand 23.5 cm [9½ in], foot 25 cm [10 in] or more would be a large frame.

Anything between these two sets of measurements would be a medium frame.

This table gives a general guide to the best weights for men and women at age 25 and over, according to frame. For girls between 18 and 25, subtract half a kilo [one pound] for each year under 25. The weights are given for persons wearing indoor clothing and shoes. Weights allow for shoes with 25 mm [one inch] heels for men and 50 mm [two inch] heels for women. If you weigh yourself in the nude without shoes you should subtract one to two kilos [two to four pounds] for women and two and a quarter to three kilos [five to seven pounds] for men.

WOMEN

metres	Height ft	in	Small frame kilos	pounds	Medium frame kilos	pounds	Large frame kilos	pounds
1.47	4	10	41-44	92-98	43-48	96-107	47-53	104-119
1.49	4	11	42-45	94-101	44-49	98-110	48-55	106-122
1.52	5	0	43-47	96-104	45-51	101-113	49-56	109-125
1.54	5	1	44-48	99-107	47-52	104-116	50-58	112-128
1.57	5	2	46-49	102-110	48-53	107-119	52-59	115-131
1.60	5	3	47-51	105-113	49-55	110-122	53-60	118-134
1.62	5	4	48-52	108-116	51-57	113-126	54-62	121-138
1.65	5	5	50-53	111-119	52-58	116-130	56-64	125-142
1.67	5	6	51-55	114-123	54-61	120-135	58-66	129-146
1.70	5	7	53-57	118-127	56-63	124-139	60-68	133-150
1.72	5	8	55-59	122-131	58-64	128-143	62-69	137-154
1.75	5	9	57-61	126-135	59-66	132-147	63-71	141-158
1.77	5	10	58-63	130-140	61-68	136-151	65-73	145-163
1.80	5	11	60-65	134-144	63-70	141-155	67-76	149-168
1.82	6	0	62-67	138-148	65-72	144-159	69-78	153-174

MEN

metres	Height ft	in	Small frame kilos	pounds	Medium frame kilos	pounds	Large frame kilos	pounds
1.57	5	2	50-54	112-120	53-58	118-129	57-63	126-141
1.60	5	3	52-55	115-123	54-60	121-133	58-65	129-144
1.62	5	4	53-57	118-126	56-61	124-136	59-67	132-148
1.65	5	5	54-58	121-129	57-63	127-139	61-68	135-152
1.67	5	6	56-60	124-133	58-64	130-143	62-70	138-156
1.70	5	7	58-62	128-137	60-66	134-147	64-73	142-161
1.72	5	8	59-63	132-141	62-68	138-152	66-75	147-166
1.75	5	9	61-65	136-145	64-70	142-156	68-77	151-170
1.77	5	10	63-68	140-150	66-72	146-160	70-78	155-174
1.80	5	11	65-69	144-154	68-74	150-165	72-81	159-179
1.82	6	0	67-71	148-158	69-77	154-170	74-83	164-184
1.85	6	1	68-73	152-162	71-79	158-175	76-85	168-189
1.87	6	2	70-75	156-167	73-81	162-180	78-87	173-194
1.90	6	3	72-77	160-171	75-83	167-185	80-90	178-199
1.93	6	4	74-79	164-175	78-86	172-190	82-92	182-204

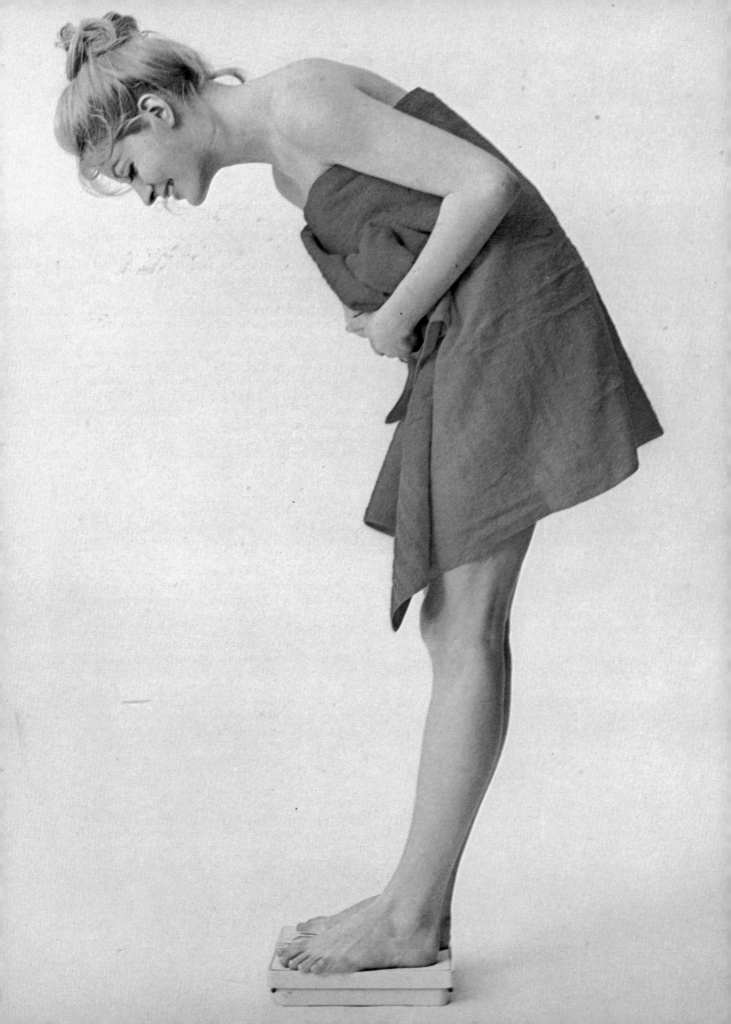

FACTS ON FAT
CONTROLLING FACTOR

What is fat? At body temperature human fat is liquid, rather like oil. It consists of glycerol (or glycerin) combined with fatty acids such as oleic, palmitic and stearic acids, which are collectively known as triglycerides. Unlike proteins and carbohydrates, fat can be easily stored in the body in cells of special connective tissue called *adipose tissue*. Most of this tissue is under the skin (about half of the body fat is found under the skin), between muscles and around the abdominal organs where it acts as an insulator and shock absorber and, most importantly, as an energy store. The composition of this energy store is approximately 85 per cent fat, 12 per cent water and two to three per cent protein. Some fat is part of the structure of body cells and cannot be used as fuel.

The fat provided by the food we eat has several functions.

It provides fatty acids essential for a great number of cell mechanisms.

It provides some of the body's energy needs.

It carries fat-soluble nutrients.

It helps the absorption of various nutrients.

It acts as an insulator against changes in temperature and as a protection for vital organs against injury.

Fat does not come only from 'visible fats' such as butter, oil and fatty meat, but also from 'invisible fats' such as milk, nuts and lean meat. Carbohydrates and proteins can be deposited as fat in the fat depots of the body.

It would seem a simple matter to cut out fat altogether when you want to slim. However, it isn't as simple as that. Some fat in the diet is essential for good health and a diet low in fat would be unpalatable and tasteless. Weight for weight, fat yields almost twice as much energy (expressed in Calories) as protein or carbohydrate, and this extra staying power seems an essential ingredient in your daily diet.

The basic figures are: one gram of protein produces four Calories; one gram of carbohydrate four Calories; but one gram of fat, nine Calories. So 28 grams or one ounce of fat gives about 252 Calories and 28 grams or one ounce of protein or carbohydrate about 112 Calories.

Fats are also the best source of certain vitamins we need. Even patients with conditions requiring minimal fat intakes do not eat a non-fat diet.

Why does fat build up?
The answer is simple. If you take in more food and drink of any kind over and above that of your daily needs the surplus is converted in your body to fat and laid down in fat cells, making them bulkier and so increasing the total adipose tissue.

At one time nutritionists believed that this adipose tissue was just so much idle padding. This is not so. Some fat from these stores is continually being used and fat from daily food replaces it. So if the amount removed is equal to the amount replaced you keep the same overall body weight. It is when the intake of energy exceeds output that the fat stores increase and body weight goes up.

The genes appear to have some influence on the relative amounts of fat in the abdomen and under the skin and the proportions in which it is laid down on the trunk and limbs. For example, there is some evidence that children in Africa, the Caribbean, and Asia have more fat on the trunk than on the limbs, compared with Western children. However, facts about the distribution of fat on the human frame are so few that experts recommend more reasearch to study the variation between individuals in the distribution of body fat between limbs, trunk and internal fat.

How much fat?
The average amount of body fat in men is 15 per cent of body weight and in women 20 per cent. But the amount can vary greatly from four per cent when a person is really almost starving to 60 per cent when the body is tremendously fat. The actual number of fat cells contained in the body is thought to be inherited; overeating later in life results in an increase in the size of these fat cells rather than an increase in the number.

Cellulite
This is one of those ideas that are so useful commercially but that have no basis in fact. 'Cellulite' is held to be a puckering of the skin, giving the effect of orange skin, over very fat parts of the body. Those who believe in it, hold that this abnormality of the skin is due to the fat being waterlogged and that it can be removed by various mechanical treatments such as massage. Conventional nutritionists and medical specialists simply do not support this idea and it has no scientific backing.

Obesity
Obesity means being fat from having eaten too much or, put more politely, an excessive accumulation of fat in the storage areas of the body. If you are more than 10 per cent above your ideal weight you are obese rather than overweight.

It is an unfortunate fact of life that fat does tend to accumulate in certain areas on some people and it is only by careful diet and exercise that this fat can be kept to a minimum.

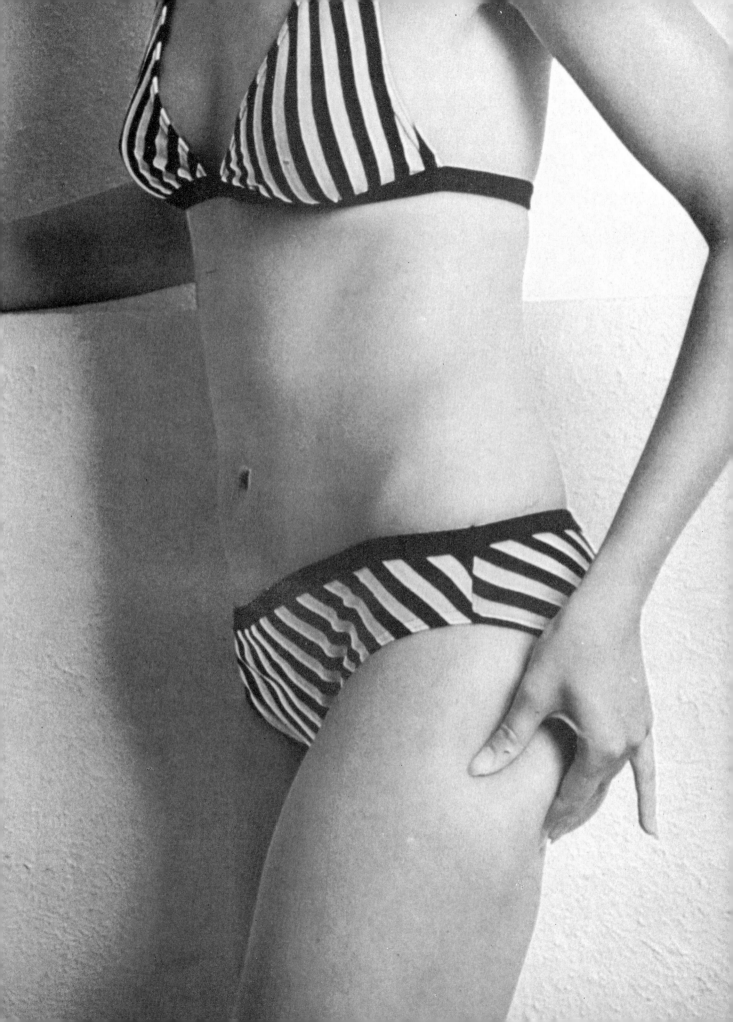

In Great Britain, for instance, there is evidence that at least 20 per cent of the population attempts to lose weight each year and that up to half the adult population is obese. Women are overweight more often than men and smokers tend to be lighter than non-smokers, though it is a delusion to assume that because you smoke you are unlikely to be overweight. Very heavy smokers, perhaps because they tend to take in calories as alcohol or sugar in tea and coffee and are less active, seem often to be heavier than the 10-15 cigarette-a-day addicts.

What causes obesity?

Obesity—being too fat—is the automatic result of taking in more food than the body can use. When energy 'in' is greater than energy 'out' the extra, whether from fat, carbohydrate or protein, is laid down in the fat cells as fat. The progress is insidious. One hundred Calories extra a day—two small boiled potatoes or a can of beer—will at the end of a year swing the needle on the scales up by 4.5 kilos [10 pounds]. Then a look in the mirror will show exactly what they have done to your shape.

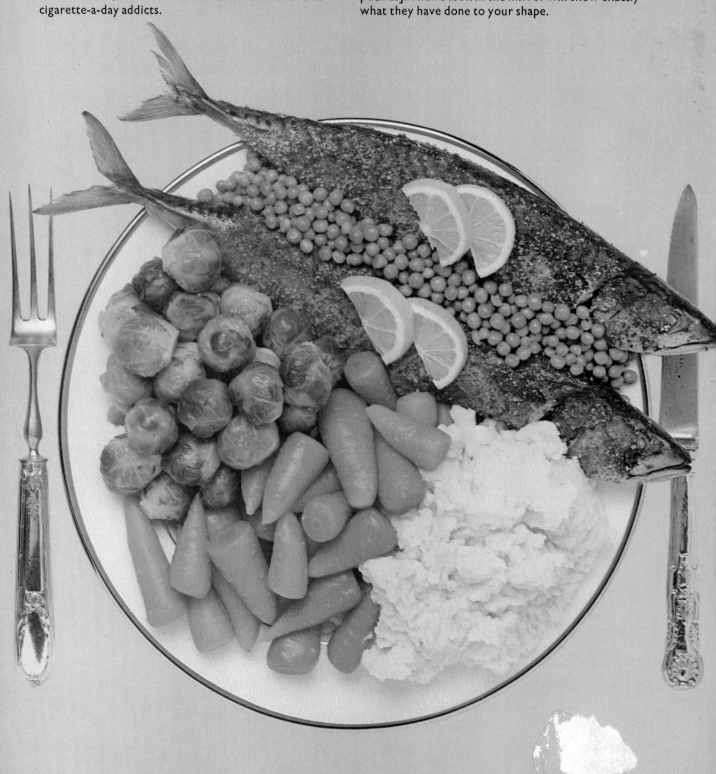

What is the cure?

If a diet gives you less energy than you need for essential bodily functions and activity at work and play, your energy store decreases, and the fat is consumed. This is the basis of slimming diets. Every gram (there are about 28 grams to one ounce) of fat burnt means nine Calories. So if you are on a diet that stipulates 1000 Calories intake a day less, your weekly loss of fat will be between 450 and 900 grams [one and two pounds] or 1.8 to 3.6 kilos [four to eight pounds] a month.

If your energy intake constantly matches your energy output, your weight will remain constant. But if, say, your energy output constantly includes half an hour's brisk walk, and you miss it one day, you will have an excess of 100 Calories to be laid down as fat.

The appetite centre

As well as daily variations, energy needs change over the years (for instance when we stop growing, or become less active) and many people seem able to change their food intake to accommodate this. What is

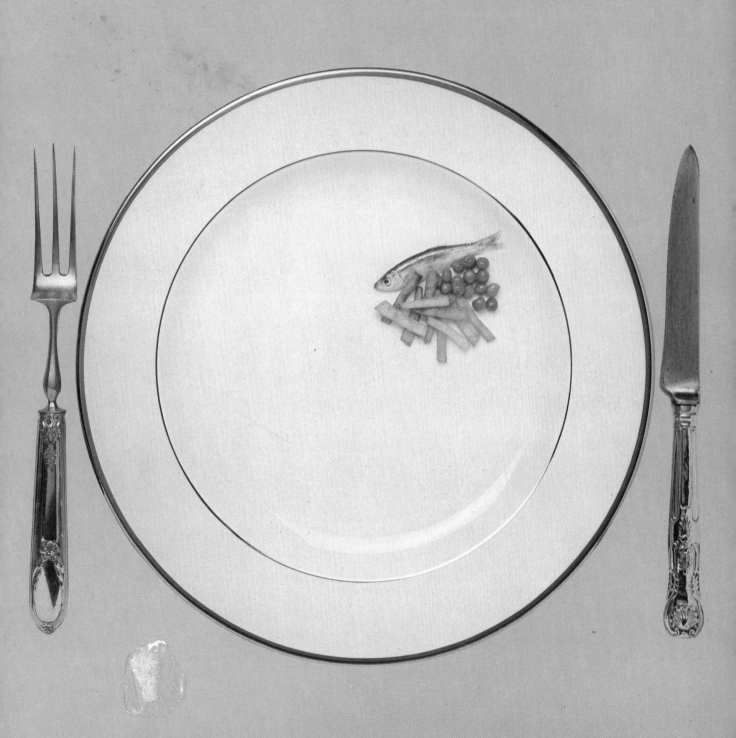

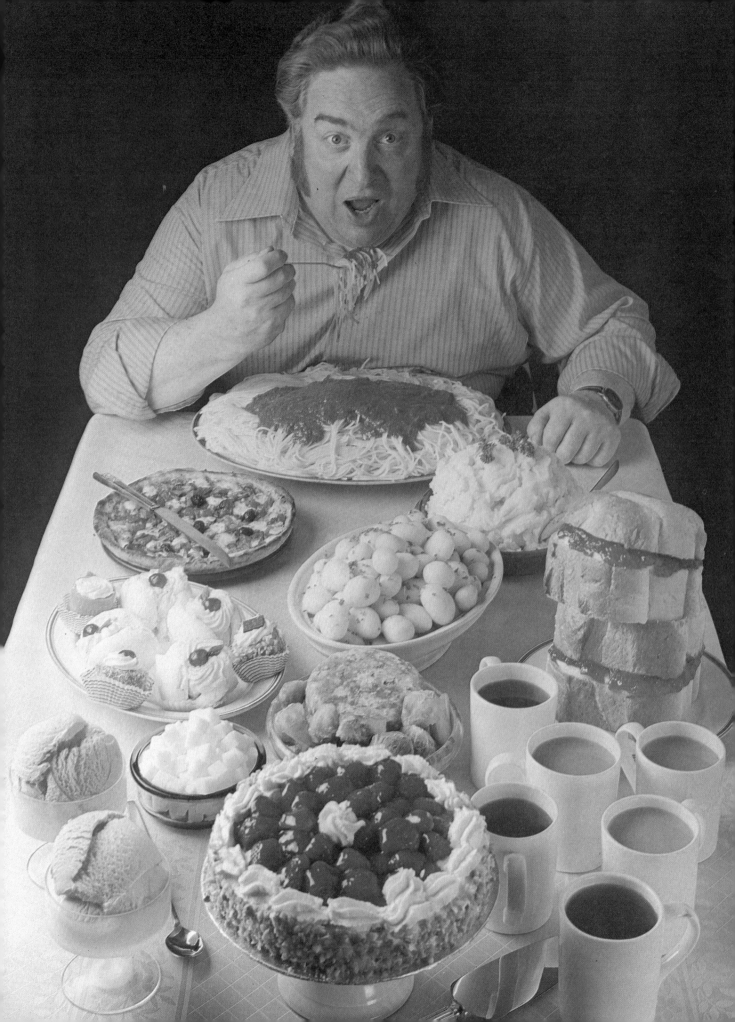

it that makes a man or woman unconsciously adapt in this way?

Like so many automatic regulators of the body (blood pressure, digestion, breathing) the appetite centre, the 'appestat', is thought to play a role in maintaining this balance. It is situated deep in the brain and is part of the hypothalamus—where many nerve centres are situated. As long ago as the turn of the century doctors observed that some patients with tumors here would develop an enormous appetite and become hugely fat.

Even stranger, scientists have more recently noticed some interesting findings with rats. Experiments in which the appetite centres were disturbed by a small operation on the hypothalamus produced voracious eating, but did not last indefinitely. After several weeks the rats reached a new peak weight and the appetite grew less and finally levelled off.

People do the same. They gain weight, reach a peak, and then remain static. The appestat seems to have set itself at a new level.

Some people seem to have the appestat all fat people envy, but how it works remains unknown, and how to make a pill that would do the appestat's work also remains a mystery.

If you are overweight, your appestat is not working properly but there are two ways in which you can help yourself. One is to get up from the table still feeling a little hungry. The other is to take exercise. The appestat in a sedentary person gradually loses its ability to control appetite accurately.

Anorexia nervosa

Anorexia nervosa is the medical name for a loss of appetite which is an illness not just a passing lack of interest in food. It should not be confused with the sometimes similar symptoms of over-enthusiastic dieting. Anorexia nervosa is usually found in young girls and is always a sign of emotional conflict. The patient refuses food but will often go to great lengths to deceive others that she *is* eating—she may hide the food she is given or otherwise dipsose of it.

Some doctors think this disturbance of appetite, like obesity itself, is becoming more common: some reports suggest that among schoolgirls aged 16 to 18, one in every 150 may suffer from it. It often begins after attempts at slimming which is more widespread among adolescent girls today than it was in the past.

Although anorexia is a dangerous disease—the patient may be so undernourished that she has little resistance to infection—treatment is essentially by psychotherapy. It is based on the theory that the rejection of food is a symbolic rejection of adult sexuality and a refusal to accept bodily and emotional changes that occur in puberty. The girl is usually of above average intelligence, hardworking, conscientious, but often at cross purposes with her family. By the time she comes to the doctor her loss of appetite is great and anything offered in the way of a decent meal makes her feel sick or throw an emotional scene.

Anorexia nervosa is best treated in hospital because a complete change of surroundings is essential for successful treatment.

Dodging the issue

It is easy for a fat person to say 'It's my glands'. If only it were true, what a simple way to lose weight: adjust the glands and the fat will slip away.

In practice very, very few fat people have trouble with their glands. And if they did, fatness would not be the main symptom to bring them to the doctor.

The sex glands, it is true, have a say in where fat is deposited. Girls become women from the influence of female hormones, one of whose actions is to lay down fat around hips and bust. And a boy who lacks male hormone lays down his fat as if he were a girl, a great embarrassment to an already plump boy. But irregularities are rare special cases, something for the textbooks and learned journals. As the old medical joke says 'the only glands involved in obesity are the salivary glands', secreting excessively to match the excessive chewing.

'It's in the family'

Big frames, heavy legs, large muscles, all these will make you weigh a lot—and they may be hereditary. But obesity means too much fat and too much fat is *not* hereditary. Identical twins, it is true, brought up separately, tend to be similar, whether it be fat, thin or average. But if they stay together, the resemblance is more marked. They pick up the same eating habits. Overweight families do tuck in and invariably into the wrong foods—the high energy ones. For good or bad, they are only happy when they have lots to eat.

So if you grew up with parents who believed that fat babies and fat children were symbols of good health, where all meals were big meals and second helpings commonplace and commendable, you have a good excuse for being obese. But it is only an excuse. You can and must break the overeating habit, despite the knowledge that a tendency to fatness does run in many families. Adopted children show this. Whereas the weights of natural children match well those of their parents, there is no such pattern between the weights of adopted children and their adoptive parents.

Fat people tend to be less active than thin people, a tendency that shows itself even before they put on weight. They sit around, take time to make a decision to move, and actually need less calories than an active person to keep their weight steady. So a fat person is really being truthful when he says 'I don't eat as much as he does but I can't get thin'.

In spite of all this, any inherited tendency to fatness does not mean that you have to be fat. Cut down on your food and you will lose weight. Exercise more and eat the same and you will lose weight (though less quickly). Cut down on your food *and* exercise more and you will lose weight more effectively.

Another excuse common among the overweight is

Re-educating your eating habits after years of high carbohydrate foods is a tremendous challenge—but the benefits of weight lost will be well worth it.

metabolism. This can be true. Some, but very far from all, fat people seem unable to metabolize fat as normally as they should, and then they cannot burn up metabolized fat as easily as others. If you are one of these people you must accept the fact that your metabolism lets you down and that you are handicapped in the slimming race. But you can still be among the winners. You can still take in less energy than you put out—despite your slightly inferior metabolism.

'I retain fluid'

For some women fluid retention is real just before menstruation and for some women on the Pill, but there is no mysterious mechanism at work in those who claim 'fluid retention' as an excuse for fatness. It is only an excuse.

The average human body contains 45 litres [47.25 quarts] of water, about three-quarters of its total constituents. Thirty litres [31.5 quarts] of this water is inside the cells; three litres [3.15 quarts] are circulating in the bloodstream; 12 litres [12.6 quarts] are in the tissues outside and among the cells. This water is all carefully balanced and an essential part of the 'interior environment'.

If you take in more water than you need you excrete more water. If you take in more salt than you need, you retain more water to dilute it. If you drink less water than you need you will be thirsty. But the healthy body keeps the balance. When you sweat a lot you lose weight because you are losing water. But you replace this when you drink again, as you have to if you are not going to become ill.

Overweight is bad for you

Slimming does more than reduce fatness: it increases healthiness. If you are overweight there are mechanical complications. You are carrying too much poundage on your frame, so some part of it has to bear the extra load.

To start on the ground, the extra weight will bear heavily on your feet, helping to flatten arches and give you flat feet. Your soles begin to ache because the ligaments in the foot are stretched when the leg muscles tire of the load.

Varicose veins appearing in the calf occur more commonly in fat people and are more difficult to treat.

Painful knees are very common symptoms in middle-aged and elderly women who are overweight. Wear and tear on the knee joint and on the hips all contribute to osteoarthritis—the joint lining begins to disappear and rough bone forms. The joint becomes painful and stiff.

Then there is backache, again a very common complaint in the doctor's surgery and made worse by the extra weight to be moved whenever the back is in action, which is most of the day. 'Disc' problems are more frequent in the overweight.

Hernias are more common in the overweight, especially the hernias of the abdominal wall where the fat carried in front strains the abdominal muscles so much that they separate enough to allow some of the intestine to protrude. And there is the hernia where

too much fat in the abdomen raises the pressure enough to push the stomach into the chest.

Too much fat around the abdomen and chest, apart from making your movements slow and ponderous can also make breathing less free. Bronchitis is often associated with overweight.

Surgeons dislike to operate on fat people. Apart from the fact that the obese are at greater risk the actual surgery is more difficult when the operational field is obscured by fat. Remember that your organs don't increase with your increased body size and weight.

All these mechanical overloadings make you easily tired, short of breath, more liable to have the general below par feeling associated with indigestion and constipation and more prone to accidents in the home and outside.

Further complications

Mechanical problems are just the start of the troubles of overweight people. High blood pressure is something like three times more common in the overweight. This is understandable if you think that a person 13 kilos [30 pounds] overweight is carrying around the equivalent of six two and a quarter kilo [five pound] bag of potatoes all day, all night, and everywhere she goes. The circulation does cope with the strains of too much work, but it will fail earlier if it is constantly under this extra pressure.

Diabetes is four times more common in the fat than in the thin, and even though it is three times as common in brothers and sisters of diabetics than in the general population, it is even more common when those brothers and sisters are fat. Too much cholesterol and other fats are found in the bloodstream of the obese. The link with increased deposits of cholesterol in the arteries and the association with heart disease are marked. Gall stones, too, are more common in the obese.

Your money and your life

Life insurance companies may ask higher premiums from the overweight. They know that they are more likely to have to pay up. Overweight people die sooner than average. If you are overweight you are therefore a poor risk. The figures are clear. Men who are 10 per cent overweight have a mortality of one fifth above the average; at 20 per cent, one third above; at 30 per cent, two fifths above. Women who are overweight are slightly less at risk but not much.

Diseases especially liable to carry them off are diabetes and diseases of the heart and blood vessels, including coronary disease. Pneumonia, cirrhosis of the liver, and accidents are lower down the list.

As Hippocrates, the Father of Medicine, said so long ago: 'Persons who are naturally very fat are apt to die earlier than those who are slender'. But the picture is not totally black.

Physicians would add a further incentive to slimmers. Lose that excess weight and blood pressure tends to come down; diabetics can sometimes do without insulin; overall mortality approaches average.

SLIMMING AIDS

There are many slimming aids available on the market but it must be remembered that all slimming aids must take second place to the slimmer's main aim: to acquire a new habit of eating where energy 'in' matches energy 'out'. Aids of any kind can offer only temporary support.

Drugs of any type should be used only on your doctor's advice. Fasting and crash diets should also not be undertaken without medical supervision.

Appetite-suppressing drugs

Amphetamines were popular once but are very rarely prescribed to treat overweight today. Doctors frown on their use because as well as suppressing appetite they also give you more energy and are 'happy' or 'pep' pills thus tempting you to become an addict, with the dangers of drug dependence and serious mental breakdown.

Phentermine and *Diethylpropion* are similar to the amphetamines but not so stimulating to the heart.

Fenfluramine suppresses appetite and also affects metabolism, helping to alter the way your body disposes of some fat and sugar.

Mazindol is another drug with the dangers of dependence. It is an anti-depressant as well as an appetite-suppressant—for a while.

Drugs that make you lose fluid

Diuretics change the balance of salt and water in the body. They force the kidney to pass more salt into the urine and more water has to go out with the salt. They do make you lose weight but again only for a while, and their true use is in diseases of the heart, liver and kidneys where fluid balance is upset.

Laxatives make you lose water from the bowels, therefore from the body as a whole giving a temporary weight loss.

Thyroid extracts are not advised; although they can work as slimming tablets they speed up all other body metabolism, not just the metabolism of food.

Bulk increasers absorb water in the stomach and make you feel full. You take them before meals and hope to eat less. Not recommended.

'Slimming' foods

There really is no such thing as a slimming food. No food has the magic ingredient that burns up fat. If it had we should all be using it. Grapefruits have been promoted mistakenly as 'fat-burners', as have lemons. It is an appealing belief that somehow, by doing no more than building a diet around grapefruit, bananas, yoghurt, rice or whatever, you can in some unknown fashion 'rid the body of impurities', 'slim away the excess fat' and so on.

The point about all 'fad' diets is that they can work because they are themselves low calorie diets. They have a place in so far as they can, if you stick to them for the recommended time, make you lose

weight. However, some of these diets can be dangerous if prolonged: eating only one or two foods means you are not getting the essential nutrients which you need for health that are provided by a well balanced diet. So use them only to make the break, so to speak, lose a few pounds and get the incentive to start a more sensible way of eating which must then become your lifelong pattern.

For people who cannot drink tea or coffee without sweetening, sugar substitutes containing saccharin are invaluable. Low calorie types of the various fruit, tonic, ginger and bitter lemon standard drinks are helpful if the slimmer really cannot do without them and change to a drink that contains practically no Calories like water, black coffee or yeast extracts. Social conventions can make it difficult to give up alcohol (as a slimmer should) but a low calorie tonic water, ice and a slice of lemon looks exactly the same as a gin and tonic.

Low Calorie products are fine to start a diet but should only be a stepping stone to new and sensible eating habits.

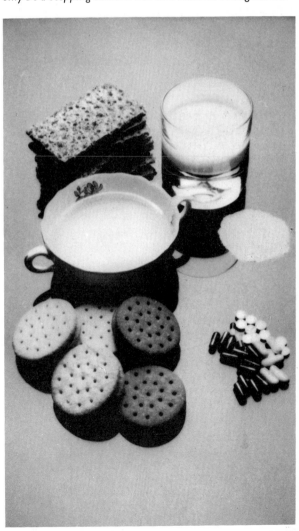

Meal replacements

Meal replacements are best used as a temporary aid to slimming and not as a permanent substitute for ordinary meals. They do not promote the essential aim of re-educating your eating habits using everyday food. These usually state the exact amount of calories and nutrients they contain.

Liquid meal replacements provide an exact number of calories with no loss of any essential nutrient and can be used as meal substitute. (They can also be used to supplement a meal for people who need extra nourishment—not a slimmer's problem.)

Solid meal replacements such as proprietary brands of slimmers' biscuits, cookies or wafers also contain a stated number of calories and nutrients. Many of them contain methylcellulose, a substance that cannot be digested so when fluid is added they make the contents bulkier giving your stomach that 'full up' feeling.

Bread and butter

Breads for slimmers are lighter slice for slice than ordinary bread but weight for weight all contain roughly equal amounts of calories. However, one slice of a slimmer's bread, because of its lightness, will contain fewer calories than a similar slice of an ordinary bread.

Low calorie margarine and butter substitutes contain about half the calories of the real thing. So does skimmed milk.

Crispbread or melba toast is lighter than ordinary bread but unless it is 'starch reduced' it contains no fewer calories than ordinary bread when matched weight for weight.

Bread contains about 50 per cent starch: if substitutes have less than this they can be labelled 'starch reduced'. In these the carbohydrate is reduced and protein substituted. Protein, although producing the same amount of calories as carbohydrate, is more satisfying and you therefore need to eat less.

Crash diets

Not to be undertaken without medical supervision and again only a temporary aid to break the overweight barrier.

Group therapy

Useful. Other people with the same problem as yourself give you the all-important motivation to carry on. They boost your willpower with pep talks, films, personal problems and helpful tips from fellow slimmers. Worth trying even if the recommended diets can be rather boring and mildly unscientific in places.

Exercise and exercisers

Exercises will certainly help burn up more calories and, if done regularly, will tone and firm muscles which will improve your shape. But remember, exercises alone will not make you shed much fat—this will only happen if the exercises are combined with a sensible and well-balanced diet.

Exercisers can also help you expend energy and thus burn up some fat. The question is whether or not they are worth the money when simple exercises needing no equipment can give just as good results if persisted with regularly. And of course any exercise would have to be regular. Just as fat is put on and muscles allowed to go slack very slowly, so a return to less fat and a trimmer figure depends on introducing new habits into your daily life. Sporadic bursts of enthusiasm will not help.

The most popular forms of exerciser, many of which can be found in gymnasiums and health salons, are the rowing machine, the bicycle, the turntable and the roller. Rowing machines and bicycles used correctly help you expend some energy but the turntable and roller very little. Don't confuse muscular development, which some exercisers promote, with energy expenditure. Such exercisers tire out your muscles long before they make you expend significant amounts of energy.

Turkish and sauna baths

As far as slimmers are concerned these are based on losing water through sweat. Boxers and jockeys are the experts here. Any weight loss is just for the bout or race. Back in everyday life the fluid has to be replaced. You do not lose body fat by this method.

Spot reducing and massage

It is an attractive and plausible idea that trained fingers, expertly kneading and slapping fat bodies, are breaking down fat and releasing it into the tissues to be carried away, never to return. The sad truth is that you can only disperse fat by burning it up. That happens only when you are taking in so few calories that the body's fat reserves are called upon.

You cannot lose weight in one spot and not another. You tend to put on fat in certain places as part of your inheritance of genes and you will find that you start to lose fat from the spot where you last put it on, but only as part of a general reduction of fat. You cannot take fat off a pot belly and not off your behind.

Mechanical massagers and vibrator belts

Mechanical massagers provide a massaging 'head' electrically driven which you apply to the part of the body from which you want to disperse fat. They cannot do this because fat cannot be released and burnt in this way.

Vibrator belts are also electrically driven and again are promoted as 'spot reducers'. You yourself are inactive while the belt vibrates. They cannot disperse fat and the only benefit is being vibrated for pleasure, if you like that sensation.

Wax

Wax preparations are also useless for dispersing fat, as are massage creams and lotions which in some unphysiological way are supposed to penetrate the skin and 'act on the metabolism'.

Weight lost through sweat is only temporary but can be a great morale booster leaving you fresh and relaxed.

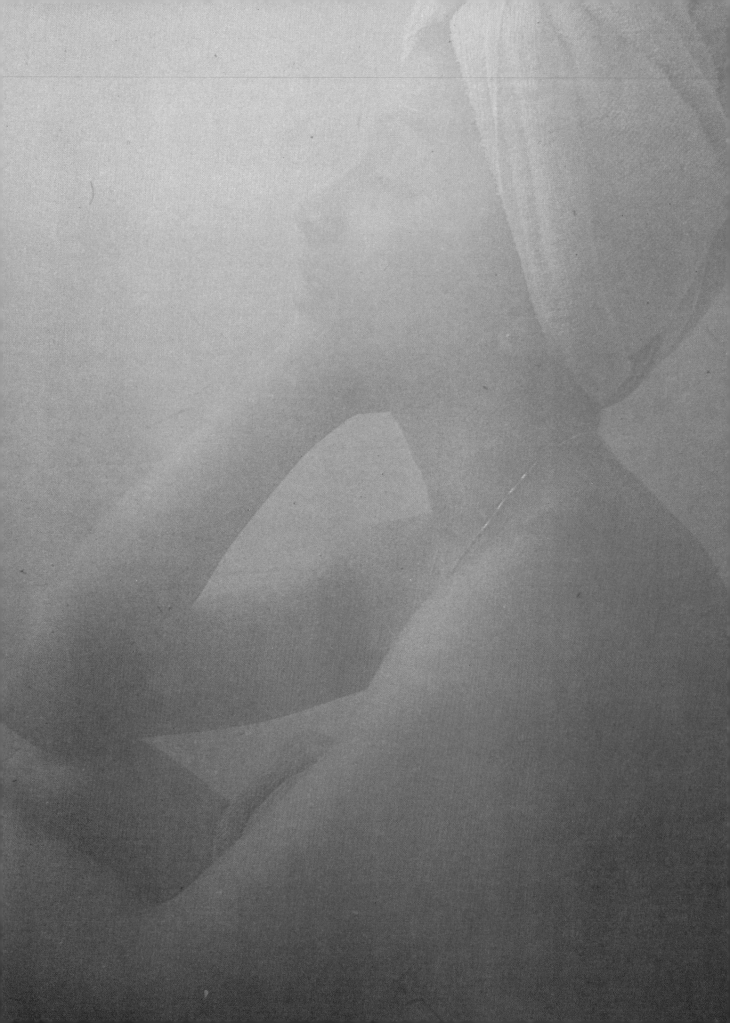

SHAPE DEVELOPMENT

Childhood fatness

It is often suggested that fat babies tend to become fat children, and many fat children become fat adults. Fat children are more common today than ever before and as weight reduction is more difficult in children than in adults it is at this time that warnings about feeding should abound. The most likely method to succeed is the restriction of carbohydrate intake, and not only in meals. Nearly all children eat too many sweets and other between-meal snacks.

A child is bound by the same energy intake rules as an adult. If the child takes in more food than is needed by the body it will be laid down as fat. Children are generally less active today than in earlier generations. Many do not walk or bicycle to school but go by car or bus instead. TV is a powerful temptation to children so that they spend more time sitting in front of it than in more active games and hobbies.

The obese adult increases in size because more fat gets laid down in the adipose tissue but the number of cells does not alter. A child, on the other hand, who is eating more than is needed can actually increase the number of cells. The consequence is that when grown-up he is more likely, because of this extra adipose tissue, to put on fat if his energy intake and energy output are not balanced.

Teenage

This is the time at which the sex hormones increase in the growing boy and girl. Girls particularly lay down the fat that emphasizes the feminnie contours.

It is particularly important not to be deceived by talk of 'puppy fat' and to assume that it will disappear as a child grows out of the teenage years. This tendency to put on fat is marked at this time of life and it is fat like any other fat.

Fat teenagers are usually less active than their contemporaries. For instance, surveys carried out in American summer camps have shown that although the fat teenagers may take part in active sports like tennis, they spend more time standing still than in running around. This of course means that, being less active, they are burning up fewer calories and unless they are eating fewer calories, the excess will be laid down as more fat.

Early adult

An uncommon age at which to begin to put on fat but men are more likely to put weight on now. It is the age at which they may give up sport, get married and settle down.

Women on the other hand are very shape conscious during this age although they may overeat by subconsciously matching food intake with their husbands.

The gradual swing to a more sedentary way of life which begins at this age also affects the working of the appetite controlling centre in the brain. This, in some

unknown way, sets the appetite so that energy intake balances energy output. But in people who take very little exercise, this mechanism seems to lose its accuracy. The result is that they find it easy to eat more than they need. The best antidote is not to give up regular daily exercise and to continue to be active, thus setting the right pattern not only for the present but also for middle and old age.

Pregnancy

Many women date the onset of fatness from their first pregnancy. 'Eating for two' is the usual reason given, but others include eating to relieve the feeling of sickness sometimes experienced in the first four months of pregnancy. This extra eating is then continued. In the second three months of pregnancy too much food will lay down fat which is masked by the natural enlargement of the womb. This fat has a special purpose: to enable the mother to breast feed her baby. If she is not going to breast feed, doctors believe that she should return to her former weight as soon as possible and not remain 30 kilos [14 pounds] (a common gain) overweight.

Middle age spread

Many women will have conquered the weight problems of successive pregnancies but found their weight steadily increasing because they were eating the children's leftovers or they were nibbling all day rather than preparing a proper meal. The middle aged woman also has the chief attendance at women's clubs, luncheons and meetings of all kinds at which carbohydrate-rich food is the stable offering, and many find they put on weight where they least want it—the waist and hips. When they begin dieting they lose their fat, not from these places, but from the neck and face, which can result in ugly folds of skin.

Many men become fat at this time simply because they find the habit of years of bread, potatoes and beer hard to drop even though they are becoming less active and more sedentary. The thickening neck, double chin and spreading waistline are there for all to see. If the appetite is really out of control protruding flesh curves from the chest to the legs.

Sensible eating is a must during middle age.

Beginning old age

As age advances all the bodily processes slow down and most people are instinctively aware that they do not need so much food and drink as they used to. But although energy needs decrease with age, the elderly still need all the nutrients and if they do not take in enough calories, cell metabolism breaks down. A balanced diet is as important at this stage of life as any other.

Sensible eating and living will keep your body looking good from childhood to adult life.

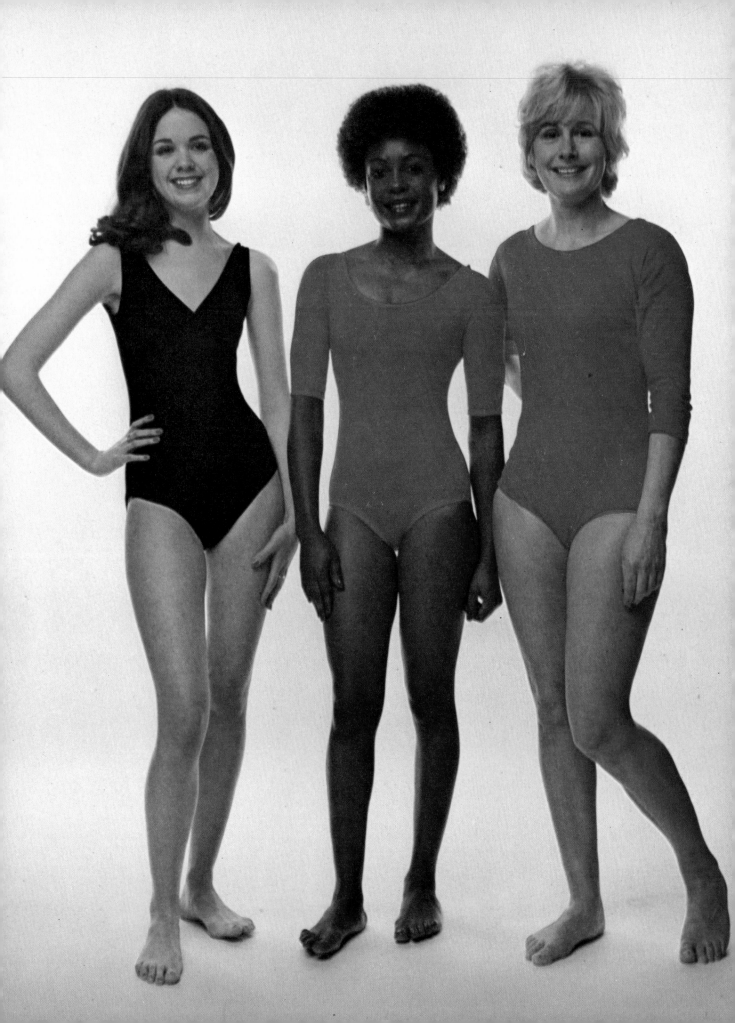

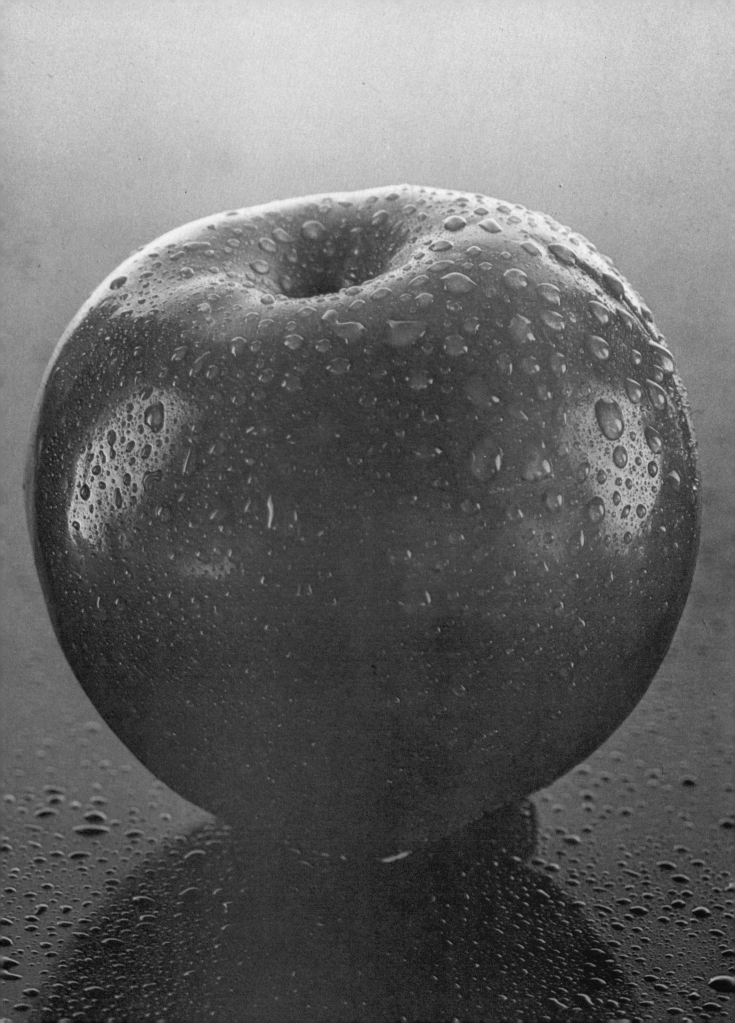

THE RIGHT ATTITUDE

Why are you fat? True there are some endocrine diseases (diseases of the ductless glands such as the pituitary) in which obesity is part of the illness, but these diseases are rare and the treatment of the obesity is the treatment of the underlying disease. For everyone else being too fat is due to eating too much for their bodily needs. So why do you eat too much? Discovering why must be your first step to a new way of eating.

Affluence

People in the Western world are better off today than they have ever been and able to buy more and richer food, particularly the sweet foods that are not essential for health and 'fast food' containing more calories than nutrients. They are also much less active than previous generations and pleasures tend to be those requiring little expenditure of energy. As part of the world you live in you cannot help but be influenced by this trend.

Way of life

Women particularly are tempted to eat too much just by being, in most households, in charge of the kitchen. When you are preparing food every day it is so easy to nibble at what you are cooking or to make yourself a 'snack'. It is the snack which is so much to blame for modern obesity. And if you have to cook a big meal for an active husband and growing children, how hard it is not to take a bigger helping yourself than you, with a relatively inactive life, really need.

Coffee mornings and similar social occasions mean more cakes, biscuits or cookies and sweets thrust in your way. 'Just this once' is a resolution seldom kept to.

However, as you go through your day, you can practise some precautions that, if they become habits, will stop you from eating too much.

Coffee break substitutes At home or in the office you can avoid the temptation to say 'yes' to cakes, biscuits or cookies by always having a supply of a low calorie food you can nibble instead—celery, a carrot, an apple or orange, or even the proverbial lettuce.

Shopping If you go shopping feeling hungry, the urge to buy more food than you need, or just a small cake or pie to eat at once, is very strong. So make a habit of shopping after you have had something to eat from your low calorie diet.

Preparing meals Take the same precautions as when shopping. If the cook is hungry when starting to cook, how easy it is to take a spoonful here and there. Much better to have a cup of lemon tea, black coffee, yeast extract, or a low calorie drink to sip instead.

Throw away Show determination to slim by clearing out 'high' calorie foods from the refrigerator, deep freeze, larder or storage shelves. Or if that seems wasteful, put them in a place where they cannot be seen.

Eating out It is not too difficult to leave your roll and butter untouched, to make one aperitif last until the first course is served, to choose melon or a clear soup followed by white fish or a grilled steak or chop, with plenty of green vegetables, and to refuse potatoes. Plenty of people do without pudding or cheese, anyway, and finish with coffee.

Liqueurs or brandy should be refused but two glasses of dry wine, red or white, can be included. Following this plan, any slimmer is eating a perfectly ordinary lunch or dinner, and not making a boring performance about dieting.

Male traps These are still the business lunch, the pub or bar and club syndrome, the rounds of drinks, and then home to a large evening meal. Admittedly, more and more men are sufficiently health conscious to go regularly to a gymnasium but the temptation of too much food and drink remains and is hard to resist when it happens every working day. The only way is to spin out the drink and quietly leave out as much as possible of energy-only food.

Alcohol Alcohol is a source of energy. Quite apart from intoxicating the brain—its best-known attribute—it is broken down in the body to be used at once as energy or stored as fat. A gram of alcohol is worth 7 Calories, more than the equivalent amount of protein or carbohydrate, so a Way of Life punctuated by regular alcoholic drinks makes the Way of Slimmer harder to follow.

Food addiction

Do you have a liking for certain types of food? Addiction is hardly too strong a word for the inability some people have to deny themselves sweet and sugary cakes, chocolates, and sweetened drinks.

Some fat people bolt their food. They do not chew it thoroughly and so eat more because the satisfaction of eating, what psychologists call oral gratification, is low.

Similar are the people who are always eating something. They need oral gratification, too, and if they are not chewing gum, drinking a cup of tea or coffee, consuming alcohol, or a sandwich, then they fill in the time with smoking. They put on weight.

The midnight visit to the kitchen is another common habit. You control your eating in the day but at night will power collapses and your hands open the refrigerator, or the biscuit tin or cookie jar for a 'snack'.

How did it happen?

Food from mother is everyone's first need. Enough food means you are not hungry. If you are hungry you are afraid that you are not loved. The association of food with affection, comfort, warmth, and love is with us for life. In childhood, food is often given or withheld as a mark of approval or disapproval. This is when good or bad eating habits are formed.

A crunchy apple is an excellent way to round off a meal.

Overeating and consequent fatness can often be traced to a lack of love at some important period in a person's life. He or she eats to stave off worry, depression, loneliness and even despair. For some people it seems to be easier to cope with difficult problems in their lives by running away from a decision and eating mammoth meals instead of trying to find a solution.

The threat before such a man or woman brings on feelings of tension and sometimes depression and the feeling (probably not conscious) that one is a helpless baby again. To be strong and invulnerable means having a big body, which means more food.

Conversely, a man or woman can unconsciously feel deserted when they have come to the end of a meal. So they go on eating as a way of warding off loneliness, not because they are hungry in the ordinary sense.
Oral gratification as a substitute for love is a common pattern found in fat people. They feel unloved and so love themselves by giving themselves food instead. They then become fat and perhaps less likely to attract the love they crave. So they eat to compensate for this lack of love and the vicious circle is complete.
Aggression can also play a part: overeating can be a way of revenging oneself on family or society. Hostility and self-hate are both shown by such people and the layers of fat could be interpreted as a symbolic way of keeping a safe distance from others.
Losing-out Fast eating and bolting of food without chewing it through, could stem from a deep fear of losing-out, of being beaten by others in the competition for food. Two reasons may be behind this trait. One is that as a member of a large family there was never really enough to eat. Another is that the family was not a happy one with rows being so frequent that the attitude to food became one of finishing a meal as soon as possible to get away before the storm burst.

Doing something about it
Psychological and emotional reasons for overeating and being fat must not deflect you from the inescapable truth that being fat means that your food intake exceeds your energy output. The decision to slim is the decision to do something about it. The first thing to decide is why you want to slim. If you have a strong aim in front of you, especially at those times like parties when Satan in the disguise of cocktails and canapes tempts you, keeping to your chosen new way of eating will be easier for you. This desire to slim must be stronger than your love of food and drink.

Vanity and better health are the best incentives to start a slimming diet. Fashion dictates that people should be slim to be sexually attractive and the majority of men and women slim with this in mind. A good time to start a diet is just before going off on holiday and on to the beach where a fat figure with loss of shape is anathema. Or you could be hoping to look your best as a bridesmaid or when looking forward to an interview for a new job. You really do feel and look better when you are not carrying around any extra pounds.

How often should you eat?
Each time you eat you increase your metabolism, so you get rid of a little more of your food over and above your energy output. This mechanism is more pronounced if you are reasonably active, and almost non-existent if you are sedentary.

The lesson for slimmers is that you will be more likely to lose weight if you have four or five meals a day rather than two. You don't alter the total daily amount of food but you do eat the total in smaller helpings more often. You then give yourself, assuming you are reasonably active, four or five little calorie-wasting boosts each day. Slimmers should incorporate this more frequent meal pattern into their way of life. But it does not mean that you eat more. The daily amount of food must remain the same.

A lot of people deceive themselves as soon as they go on a diet, particularly when they get to that stage when weight loss slows down. This can happen as early as the second week. Weight has gone down quite nicely because the stores of glycogen (carbohydrate stored mainly in the liver) are easily used up, and together with this goes quite a lot of water. But it takes twice as long to lose half a kilo [one pound] of fat as it does to lose the same amount of glycogen. Little water is lost from the fat cells and the temporary halt discourages many slimmers.

Deception can also take the form of forgetting about snacks eaten or calories wrongly counted. So diets that limit the foods you can eat, rather than the amount (like the low carbohydrate diet) are better for these absent-minded slimmers. You can't deny that you have eaten a bar of chocolate.
If you are forgetful or inclined to cheat, you will find it easier to keep track of your diet if you buy a separate diary and each day write down exactly what you eat.

Making a performance
Slimming is easier for some people when they can make a ritual out of their diet. This could include special care and faddiness when shopping. If you are allowed, say, six pieces of crispbread a day or one slice of wholemeal bread, finding the best and most exclusive brands could enable you to take pride in eating only your allowance of this expensive food. And if you enjoy cooking, now is the time to experiment with new ways of preparing the meat, fish, vegetables and eggs your diet prescribes. And you can be meticulous in planning weekly menus.

Alcohol
Alcohol is a food and provides something like 200 Calories per 28 grams [one ounce] but, quite apart from the calorie content, you should be careful of it: under its influence you lose some self-control, enough perhaps not to resist food you have pledged yourself not to have. Remember all those parties when you dug into the peanuts and crisps after a glass or two of whisky or wine.

Re-educating eating habits means declining that high Calorie cream gateau for a low Calorie fresh fruit dessert.

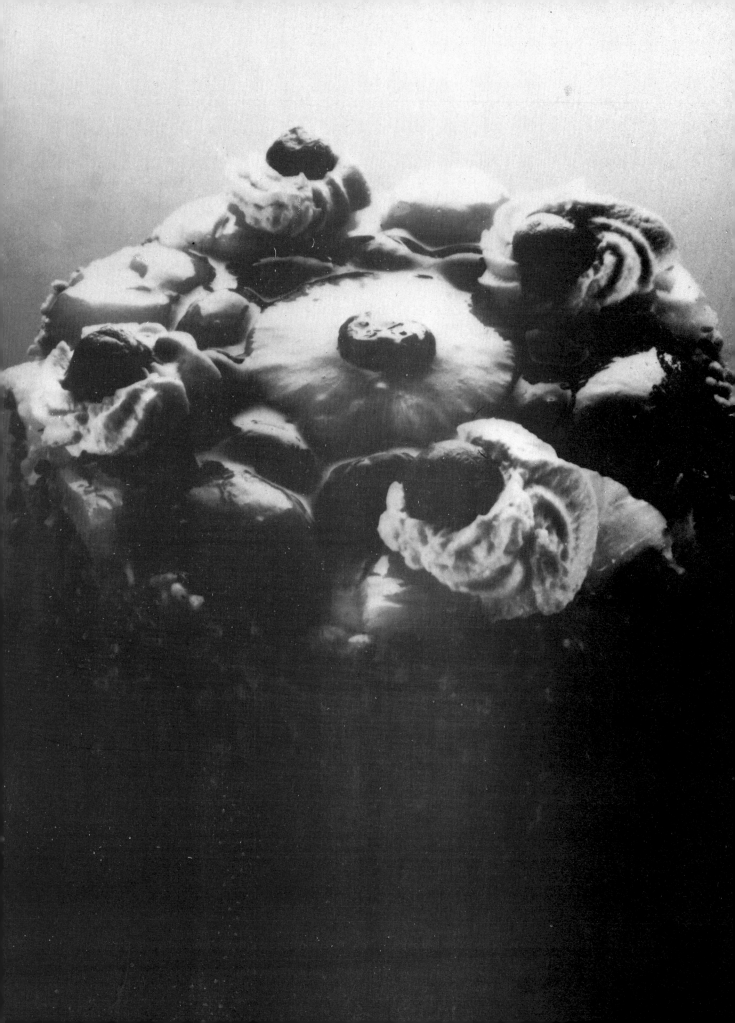

HEALTHY LIVING

Being the best weight and shape for the body you have is only part of healthy living, although a vital part. You are well on the way to having a positive attitude to maintaining that weight and to keeping fit. You have got into the habit of 'thinking thin' and looking and feeling better as a result.

Doctors today, as well as the general public, are turning back to the old belief in fresh air and exercise as essential for good health. This belief, of course, has never been completely dismissed but its revival matches the concern experts and lay people feel about the dangers of the sedentary life many of us now lead.

So many people are becoming less active. They go to work by car, train, or bus instead of walking or bicycling. They sit down for the best part of their day at work instead of having to move about and at home slump in front of the television. If you are relatively inactive in this way you are likely to gain weight because you are not using very much energy.

You may protest that the amount of weight lost by regular exercise is so small as to be not worth worrying about. This is not entirely so. For instance a half-an-hour's slow walk a day would use up the equivalent of 100 Calories and so long as you ate no more than usual you would lose 225 grams [half an ounce] in weight. Exactly, you might reply, not worth worrying about. But that regular daily loss, means about 450 grams [one pound] lost over a month, or about 5.5 kilos [twelve pounds] in a year—a worthwhile objective. And this does not include the other benefits of regular exercise, the pleasure of using your muscles, lungs and heart more fully than before, the feeling of well-being, the toning of muscles, the sounder sleep.

Exercise a substitute for diet?
A common belief among the 'no-nonsense' school is that if you ride, play tennis, golf, squash or even cricket, you can eat what you like without getting fat. Not true. It is as false as the idea that exercise only makes you eat more.

What you need is the right blend of both dieting and exercise if you want to lose weight most effectively and then to lead a healthy life. The secret here is not to rush things. Just as your pattern of eating takes time to adjust to—after all you took years to put on weight —so exercise should gradually become a regular, reasonable part of every day life. Integrate it with everything you do in your daily routine. A few very simple habits to acquire are: to climb the stairs for three or four floors instead of using the lift or elevator.

Don't just sit at your desk but move about at work as much as you can.

Walk to and from work or, if that is not practical walk to the next station or bus stop.

Use a bicycle as much as possible. If you usually go to the shops by car, use your bike instead.

Learn to stand and sit well and make it a habit. So many people slouch. If you sit upright and hold yourself up when standing or walking you will be surprised how much this improves your shape. It's a mild form of exercise too.

Slack muscles, especially abdominal ones, can be strengthened by exercises. They will regain their tone and you will regain your shape: a previously protruding belly could soon become flat again.

Try this simple exercise while sitting at your desk or waiting for a bus or train:

Breathe out as fully as you can so that your lungs seem empty. Then slowly draw your abdominal muscles upwards and backwards as far as they will go towards the spine. Hold this hollow you have made for about six seconds and let your muscles relax slowly. Breathe in, and then repeat as often as you like. Rounding your shoulders slightly and leaning forward slightly will help you to get maximum contraction from the muscles.

Health farms
Health farms have grown more popular as spas have declined and today there are many to choose from.

Health farms are really for the weak-willed and they are expensive. If you feel like being pampered for a week or two in peaceful surroundings with the object of getting back in trim, one of these establishments is the place for you.

They offer a regular routine of dieting, baths, exercises, massage and all the luxuries a tired body will welcome. You eat very little, and at the end of your stay will almost certainly have lost quite a bit of weight and feel rejuvenated. However, this weight loss will be replaced unless you keep to a well balanced diet.

Slimming magazines and clubs
Strengthen your resolve by reading expert advice and life stories of successful slimmers. Several of these magazines run slimming clubs and have branches in most countries and large towns. Each have their rules and entrance and membership charges.

Health foods
Unless you happen to prefer a 'health' food product to the others available in ordinary shops and stores, there is no special 'slimming' value in them.

A 'health' food is grown or produced on land where no artificial fertilizer is added and is 'whole' or 'natural'. This means that nothing is added or taken away from the food, and it contains no added chemicals. However, there is no evidence that health food is better for you and you should remember that because a food is 'natural' you are not necessarily going to eat it with impunity. Just because it is a health food it isn't necessarily non-fattening!

Keeping your body in good shape calls for healthy outdoor exercise as well as a balanced diet.

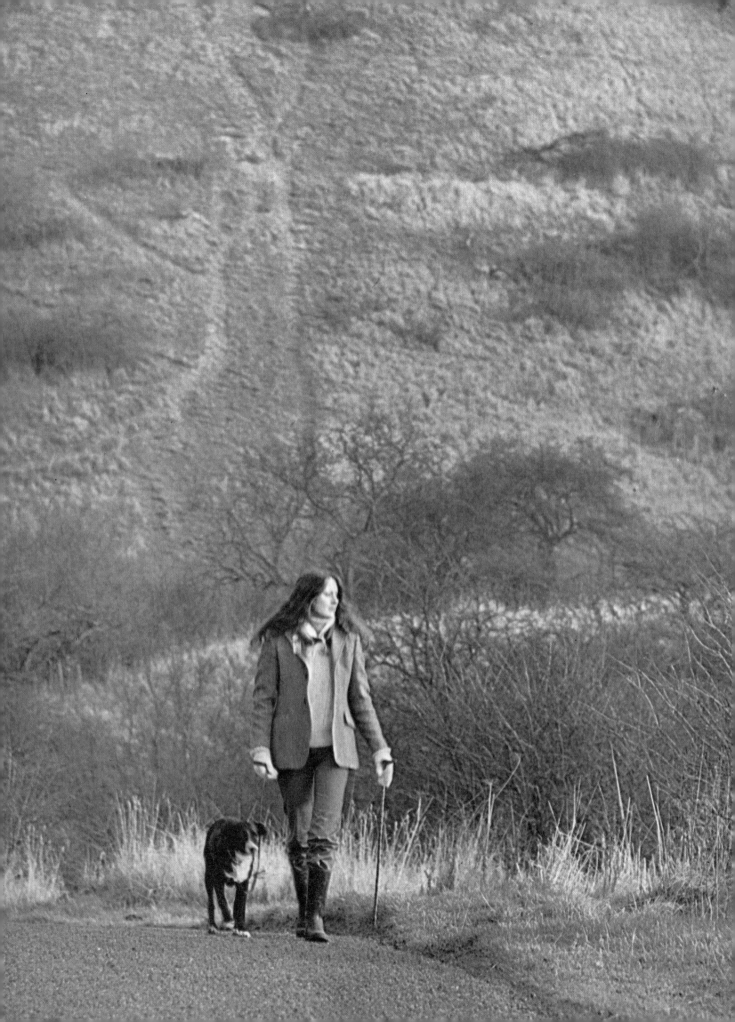

SPORTS

No slimming campaign is complete if it does not encourage sensible exercise as a daily feature to match new eating habits. Sport offers a tremendous variety of ways of taking exercise.

Our bodies are built for movement, for muscles to contract and extend, for joints to flex.

The body's autonomic nervous system reacts to exercise in the same way as it does to a 'fight or flight' emergency. Hormones release extra fat from the body's fat stores and divert this fuel to muscles that need it. This is done by dilating the blood vessels to the muscles and narrowing those to the digestive system, which quiets down during an emergency. This is the body's way of preparing itself for aggression and competition, for 'fight'. 'Flight', ie anxiety and uncertainty, stimulates adrenaline to release glucose into the bloodstream and the heart beats quicker so that this fuel supply can also reach the muscles. The lungs take in more oxygen to burn it. And the sweat glands go into action to help cool the body.

In our active life these stress reactions are often not followed by any physical activity. We are tense and frustrated, the energy is unused and blood pressure rises. Exercise protects us against this. It uses up the extra fuel and prevents much of the rise in blood pressure by forcing blood to the widened vessels in muscles needing the extra energy. In the widest sense exercise lessens stress, not only at the time but for some days after.

Cycling, swimming, dancing, skiing, skating, golf, and, though not strictly sports, gardening and walking, are suitable for most people, without regard to age or sex.

This is because all use the majority of muscles, which guarantees a relatively large energy output with a moderate amount of exertion. Running and jogging and most ball games belong to this group though not so widely recommended for everyone.

Riding, body-building, gymnastics, involve smaller groups of muscles. Exertion is relatively great and the expenditure of energy relatively low.

Which sport?

Swimming is considered an ideal exercise for all ages. It uses most muscles and is smooth and rhythmic as well as offering many different strokes.

Squash, like swimming, is easy for city dwellers to take up because courts are readily available as are swimming pools. Very heavy activity so should not be played strenuously by the unfit.

Ping-pong, again, is easy for the city dweller and gives light to moderate exercise.

Archery is suitable for all ages and a sport you can play into old age. Quite a lot of standing about.

Skiing is a sport the middle aged and some elderly practised skiiers can also enjoy. Moderate exercise when a combination of downhill skiing and being hauled back up a slope. (Cross-country skiing as native to Scandinavia is more arduous.)

Golf gives you exercise that is mostly walking, as long as you do walk and don't use a cart. It can vary depending on how fast you go round the course including waiting for your opponent to play his stroke and find lost balls. A good golfer will play less strokes than a novice.

Gardening is an ideal exercise for the not so young since a gardener can choose how energetic he wants to be and can do light, moderate or heavy work.

Walking is perhaps the basic 'sport' and a good first step to keeping fit as it uses most muscles. Again, the walker can choose his own pace.

Jogging is a good exercise, but it is important not to overdo it. The best pace is one that allows you to talk easily to anyone who happens to be beside you.

Cycling, like swimming, is smooth and rhythmical and the cyclist can choose his own pace.

Important

Although physical activity carries less risk to health than inactivity, anyone doubtful about his or her health should consult a doctor before embarking on any strenuous sport he or she is unused to.

Calorie expenditure in some everyday sports

The figures given indicate the Calorie expenditure per minute by men. Women expend approximately one Calorie less per minute. These figures are average since no two people are likely to expend the same amount of energy. One may run all over the court in a tennis match, while the other stands at the net and volleys every shot, moving much less.

The figures are deceptive in another way. Squash, for example, demands more energy than tennis, but a tennis match is likely to last longer with the result that the total amount of energy used could be greater.

Cricket	2.5 to 3.7 to 6.6
Sailing	2.5 to 3.7
Trampoline	2.5 to 3.7
Archery	2.5 to 5.2
Fishing	2.5 to 5.2
Croquet	2.5 to 3.7
Bowls	2.5 to 3.7
Golf	2.5 to 7
Tennis	5.2 to 6.6
Squash	7.9 snd over
Badminton	3.7 to 5.2
Surfing	3.7 to 5.2
Rowing	5.2 to 7.9 and over
Underwater swimming	5.2 to 6.6
Swimming	5.2 to 7.9 and over
Climbing	5.2 to 7.9 and over
Skating	5.2 to 6.6
Skiing	5.2 to 7.9 and over
Basketball	5.2 to 6.6
Football	5.2 to 7.9 and over
Hockey	5.2 to 6.6
Rugby	6.6 to 7.9 and over
Fencing	5.2 to 6.6
Karate	5.2 to 6.6
Wrestling	7.9 and over
Boxing	7.9 and over

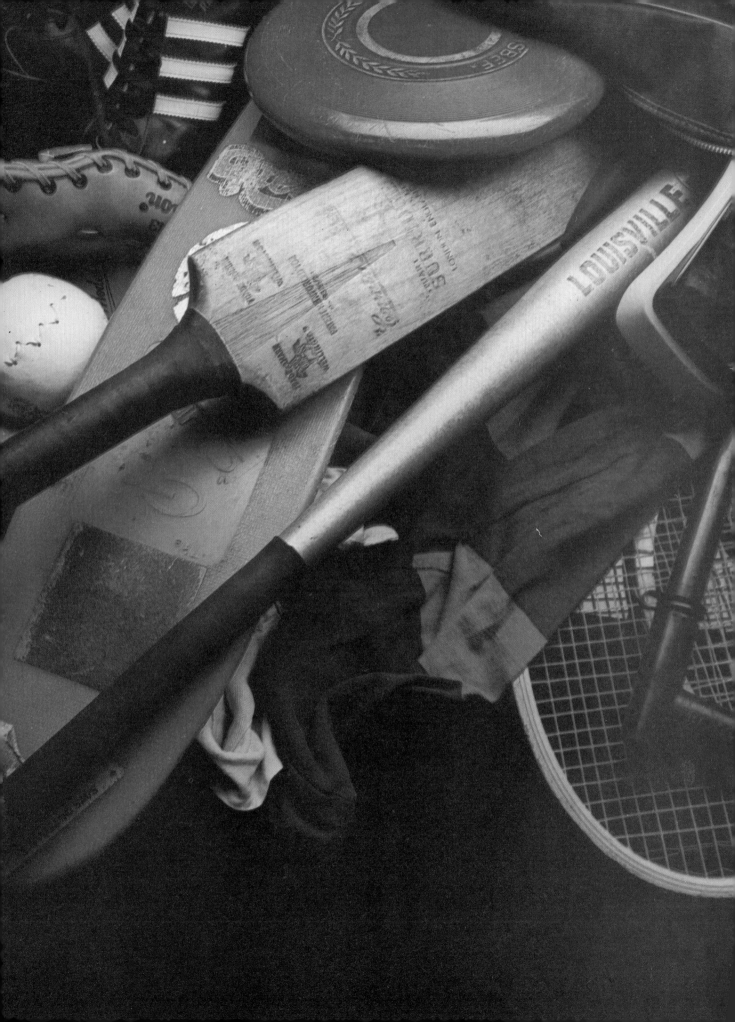

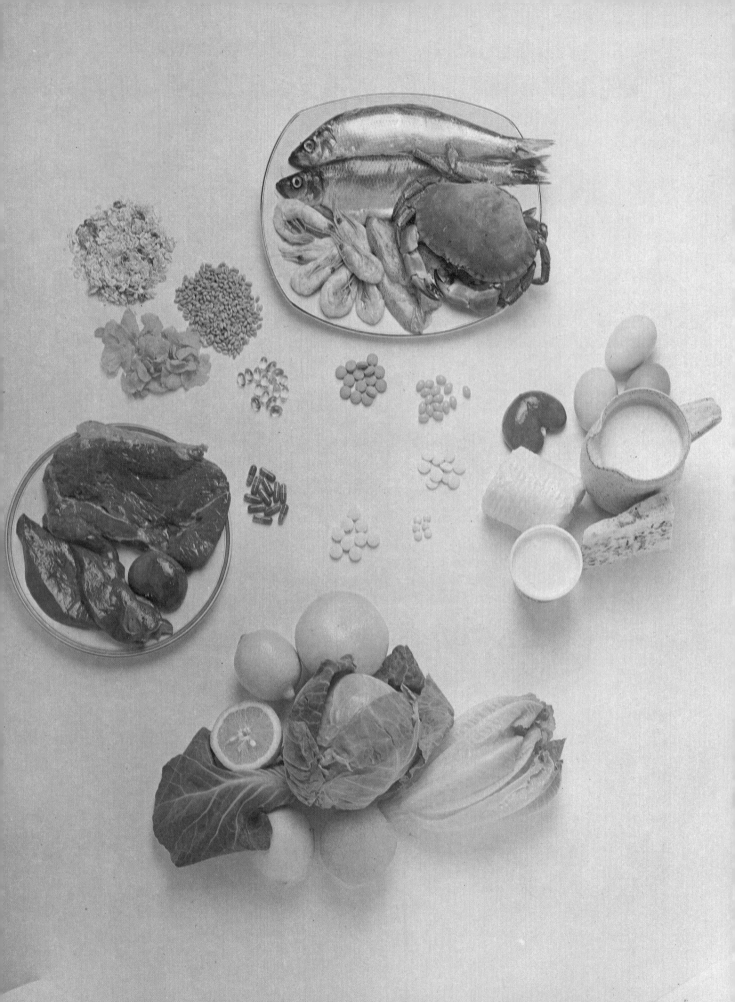

FACTS ON FIGURES
NUTRITIONAL NEEDS

Nutrients are substances present in food that are vital for all-round health. They have two main functions. One is to provide energy: the other is to promote growth, maintain and repair body tissues and cells, and to regulate body chemistry. All nutrients can be found in food though not all foods, by any means, contain all nutrients—hence the importance of a balanced diet.

The nutrients and energy you need depend on your size, sex and occupation. But even so, people do vary from one another in their needs although seeming to be so alike. And the amount you need of any one nutrient is influenced by the rest of the food you are eating. The reason is that the efficiency with which a nutrient is used by the body is affected by the quality and type of your whole diet.

Official lists and tables and charts of daily nutritional needs recognize the facts when calculating their figures. They also insist that the recommended intakes are for healthy people and not those needing special diets, and that there is no benefit in eating more than the recommended amounts.

You need energy for the various bodily activities, both voluntary, such as exercise, and involuntary, such as digestion, and to provide heat to keep body temperatures constant.

Energy comes from protein, fat, carbohydrate and alcohol but they need the presence of vitamins and minerals to release it. The kilocalorie (Calorie for short) is the term used to measure energy released.

The body cannot grow unless it has enough nutrients. That is, extra on top of those needed to supply energy and basic maintenance.

Body tissues, bones, deposits of fat, blood cells, plasma, hair, nails are continuously being replaced. The bigger the body the greater the amount of replacement needed.

The 'internal environment' of the body depends on the presence of vitamins, enzymes, minerals and hormones. Minerals and vitamins are nutrients. Hormones and enzymes are manufactured within the body from nutrients in food.

The five types of nutrients needed by the body in addition to water and oxygen are:

Protein Essential for growth, repair and maintenance

There is a wide range of vitamin supplements available on the market but most people are supplied with sufficient amounts through eating a properly balanced diet. Iron in meat and eggs. Vitamin E in wholewheat and grain cereals. Kelp in sea foods. Vitamin B complex in dairy produce and kidneys. Calcium in milk, cheese and yoghurt. Vitamin A in vegetables, offal and diary products. Vitamin C in green vegetables and citrus fruit.

of body tissue and as the basic substance from which hormones and enzymes, which aid in energy production, can be built. Protein left over after basic needs have been met can be broken down and provide a source of energy if needed, or it can be converted to carbohydrate and fat and stored for future use.

Fats are a good source of energy and also carry the fat-soluble vitamins A and D. It is necessary to have deposits of fat to protect the vital organs, and beneath the skin to preserve body heat.

Carbohydrates provide energy as their main job. If not used, they are stored as glycogen to be an energy reserve or are converted into fat and stored in the adipose tissue.

Minerals. These do three separate jobs:

In the body tissues minerals such as phosphorus, iron, zinc, copper and sulphur are found in muscles, blood and liver and are essential in the processes which release and use energy.

In the body fluids the most important minerals are salt and potassium which play a leading part in keeping the body fluids constant.

In bones and teeth calcium, phosphorus and magnesium are the predominant minerals. Teeth and bones are solid compared with the blood and soft tissues and are chiefly made of minerals.

Other minerals that play a part in nutrition are fluorine (for tooth enamel), iodine (for the thyroid hormone controlling the rate of metabolism), and zinc cobalt and manganese.

Vitamins are vital for the unending chemical reactions of the body metabolism. These are grouped as follows:

Vitamin A (Retinol) is needed for normal eyesight, growth and a healthy skin. A deficiency of vitamin A could result in inflammation of the eyes and premature ageing of the skin.

Vitamin B Not one vitamin but a complex of several, all of which carry out vital cell metabolism and many are involved in energy release.

Vitamin C Needed for the functioning of the connective tissues and intercellular substance. If Vitamin C is lacking the blood vessels bleed readily giving rise to scurvy. The body's need for vitamin C is increased when it is tired or under stress.

Vitamin D Fat-soluble and essential for healthy teeth and bone. It helps absorption of calcium and phosphorus from the intestine and is vital for the movement of calcium from the inside to the outside of bones during growth. Vitamin D is also made by the action of sunlight on the skin. A lack of vitamin D can result in weak, brittle bones, painful joints and rickets.

Vitamin E is found chiefly in vegetable oils, cereals

and eggs as it is fat soluble. It has no known function in man, although it may be vital for healthy red blood cells.

Vitamin K Fat-soluble and necessary for the formation of an enzyme, thrombin, which is essential for blood clotting. It is given to patients who are liable to bleed heavily when vitamin K is poorly absorbed. It is also sometimes given to prevent bleeding in new-born babies.

The body's need for water
Water makes up 70 per cent of the body and shares in many of the metabolic reactions constantly going on. Each cell is surrounded, for instance, by fluid of an exact chemical content, and water forms the basis of this fluid. It also holds and carries materials in the intestine, in the blood and in the cells.

Water is used in many of the changes taking place in the food during digestion and later when the products of digestion are absorbed from the intestines. It is the predominant compound in human diet and essential for keeping temperature stable.

In a temperate climate, for example, the body needs about three litres [5 pints] of water a day, that is the average amount of daily loss. You would need to actually drink about one and a half litres [two and a half pints] daily, the remaining one and a half litres [two and a half pints] would come from your daily food intake and from the by-products of metabolizing it.

Which food, which nutrient?
You cannot buy and eat food on the assumption that each separate food contains only one of the nutrients or, for that matter, all of them. Most foods contain one predominant nutrient and smaller amounts of others. You can group the food we depend on into animal and

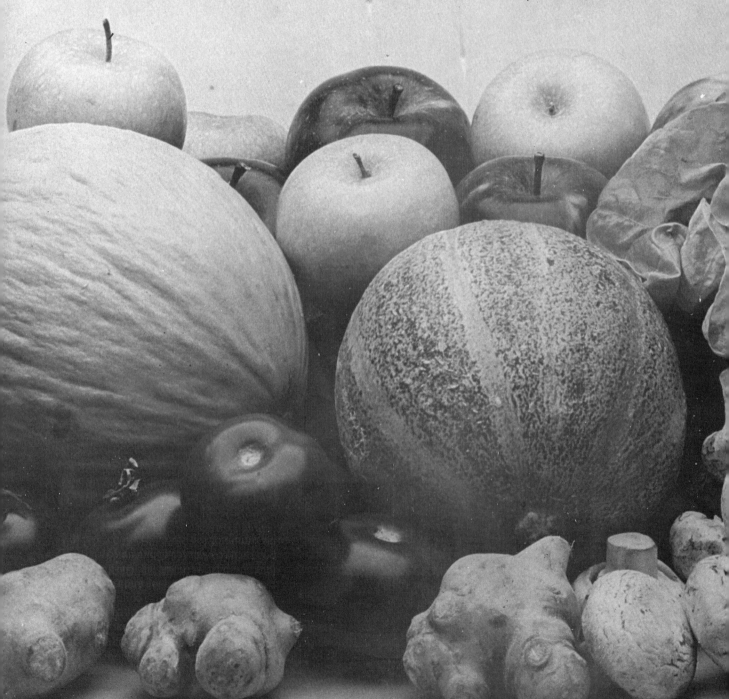

plant food or into four main groups:

Meat, fish, eggs, nuts, legumes
This group is the main protein source needed for growth and maintenance. These foods also supply iron and vitamins of the B group. Eggs and liver are good sources of vitamin A. The food from this group also contains a significant amount of fat, except for dry beans and peas.

Milk and cheese
High in calcium and phosphorus needed for growth and maintenance of the bones; milk also provides significant amounts of protein, vitamin A, D and some B group.

The bread-cereal group
Cereal forms a major part of man's diet, mainly in the form of wheat products such as bread and flour. They are a good source of B group vitamins, contain some protein, fat and iron and are good sources of energy.

When the outer coat of wheat is removed some of the valuable nutrients go with it, so in many countries the law insists on addition of iron and B group vitamins to white bread.

Fruit and vegetables
Good sources of vitamins and minerals and important as dietary fibre in the diet. Fruit is the main source of vitamin C, particularly oranges, lemons, grapefruit and, best of all, blackcurrants. Green vegetables carry vitamin C and some other vitamins and minerals in their leaves. Swedes [rutabagas] and turnips are also good sources and some is also found in potatoes. But root vegetables are mainly a source of carbohydrate. Vegetables like rhubarb and celery contain a lot of indigestible carbohydrate in their stems.

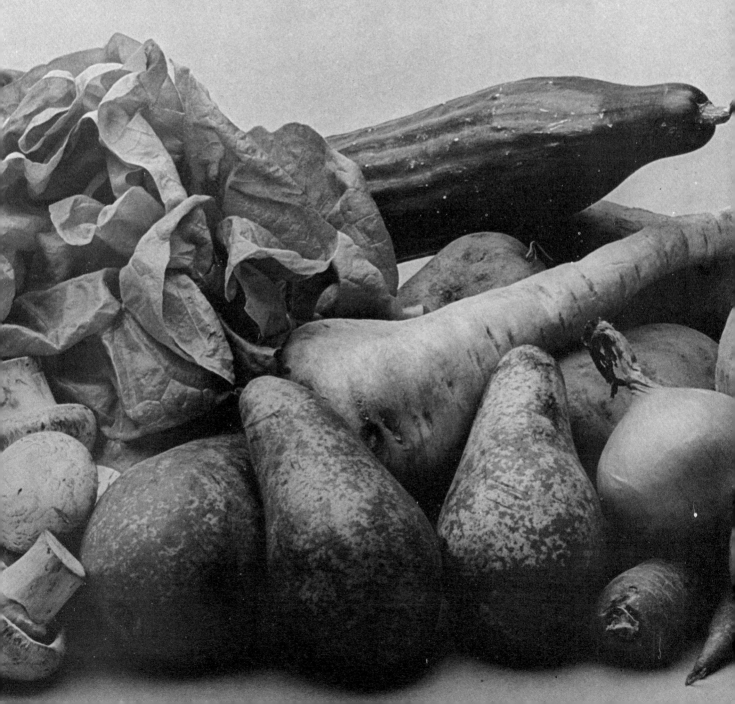

WHAT IS ENERGY?

To talk of 'burning', 'taking in' or 'using up' calories is misleading. Although easy ways of specifying the amount of food eaten and energy expended during activity, all these phrases suggest that a calorie is part of food. It is not. A calorie is a unit of measurement, an expression of energy which can be obtained from food and is vital for maintaining life. You cannot eat a calorie, or buy any food or drink that contains it, as you can proteins or vitamins.

A calorie is a measurement of heat, a form of energy, produced when food is chemically burnt as it is when metabolized in the body. The definition of a calorie is 'the amount of heat needed to raise the temperature of one gram of water by one degree centigrade'. But in the science of nutrition it is more convenient to use the kilocalorie, the same as 1000 Calories (with a capital C) which is defined as 'the amount of heat needed to raise the temperature of one kilogram or one litre of water by one degree centigrade'.

Calories are calculated from the amount of oxygen used to consume chemically the body's fuel taken in as food (one litre of oxygen used to burn food gives about five Calories of heat), or directly by measuring the amount of heat the body gives out. So when the Calorie content of food and drink, and the Calories used in various forms of bodily activities are talked about, they are derived from these measurements.

To make slimming more confusing the Calorie is now being dropped and some nutritionists are in favour of the Joule which is the unit of all forms of energy instead of just the unit of heat. However, so long as the slimmer understands that both the Calorie and the Joule are different methods of measuring *energy value*, we will continue to use the Calorie. Perhaps the word 'energy' needs defining.

Energy in body metabolism is not the same as 'pep' or vigour or strength. It is chemical energy derived from the action of oxygen on food once it has been digested and absorbed. Protein, carbohydrate and fat, some or all of which are contained in every food, supply this biological fuel. Thus all food, our body fuel, can be burnt with the same end result—carbon dioxide and water—as when a piece of coal is burnt. If, for example, a scientist burns glucose or wheat in a laboratory experiment, a similar amount of energy is produced as if a man had consumed it. The difference is that, in the body, the energy is released only gradually in a series of tiny steps. These steps are controlled by the enzymes, helped by minerals and vitamins. The tiny amount of energy released at each step is used for a special purpose, say, to build up a body protein.

If burnt in the ordinary way, glucose or wheat would need a tremendous amount of heat to catch alight and release its energy.

What happens in the body is that the red blood cells in the lungs take up oxygen from the air and carry it to where it unites with the energy-supplying nutrients the end products of digestion. This changes the chemical nature of the nutrient and at the same time releases energy in the form of heat, mechanical energy, electrical energy or chemical energy (all energy can be converted to any other form of energy).

Mechanical energy Complicated changes when glucose is chemically burnt convert chemical energy into mechanical energy so that muscle fibres contract and produce movement.

Heat energy Mechanical energy is partly concerned in giving off heat. So when the body muscles are working the body as a whole becomes warmer. This is in addition to the constant mechanical energy used in breathing, the circulation of the blood and other involuntary activities.

Electrical energy Small amounts of chemical energy are used continuously for conversion to electrical energy. The heart discharges electricity, a fact made use of in electrocardiography, and so does the brain, whose waves can be recorded.

So energy can be defined as the ability to do the body's work. That is to maintain life (the basic functions such as breathing and digestion), to provide for voluntary activities (those under our direct control such as walking or running), and for times when extra energy is needed (when children are growing and women are pregnant or breast feeding).

Energy expenditure and body size

The heavier a person, the more energy he needs. The energy used in walking, for example, is in proportion to the body weight of the person. For specific activities the relationship is close. But the relationship is not close between the *total* daily activity and body weight. The reason is thought to be that heavy people are less active and are sluggish, compared with lighter people. So when working out the energy expended by groups of people in different occupations, it is the occupation that matters rather than the weight of the individual involved.

In the Western world most people get their energy from food in these proportions: protein 10 to 15 per cent; fat 30 per cent; carbohydrate 65 per cent. A daily average for each person's diet is 85-113 grams [three to four ounces] of protein, 113 grams [four ounces] of fat and 425 grams [15 ounces] of carbohydrate. Most of this food goes to supply energy with a relatively small amount being used for growth, reconstruction and replacement of tissues.

Weight for weight fat has the greatest energy value, 28 grams [one ounce] giving about 250 Calories. 28 grams [one ounce] of carbohydrate gives about 112 Calories and protein gives just slightly more than carbohydrate.

Whether active or asleep, the body is using energy, and one of the best ways of making full use of the body's energy resources is through vigorous physical exercise.

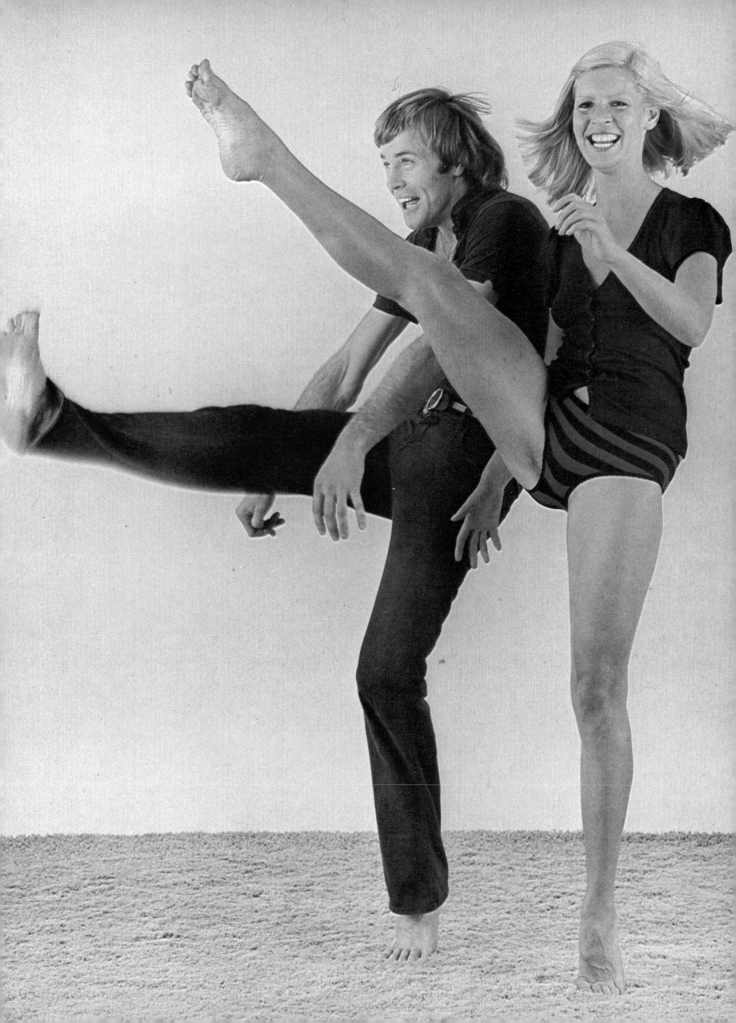

ENERGY NEEDS

A person needs energy to maintain life, for work and play and for the special needs already mentioned. More energy taken in than needed is laid down as fat.

Maintaining life This consumes well over half the average man or woman's energy. Women have a lower basic energy expenditure than men partly because they are smaller, partly because they have less muscle and more fat. Children's basic metabolism in proportion to their size is greater than that of grown-ups, but in the elderly it is less. A big man needs more energy for his basic metabolism than a small man.

What is this basic metabolism? It is the sum of all the building-up and breaking-down processes going on in the body, awake or asleep. Doctors call this the basal metabolic rate (BMR) and measure this 'ticking over' while a person is lying down relaxed, comfortable and warm. Included in the BMR are the heart beating, the lungs taking in and pushing out air, the movement of the stomach and bowels, the work of the brain and the production of hormones.

People vary from one to another in their energy needs for basic metabolism because some bodies work more efficiently or tick over faster or slower. But an *average* energy need for an *average* man is 3000 Calories a day. He needs about one Calorie a minute to maintain life. A woman needs slightly less.

When a person engages in any sort of activity the demand for energy is bound to increase.

Activity in work and play Scientists have measured the amount of energy expended in all kinds of activities. Again, as with the BMR, the figures are average because individual efficiency varies from person to person. A skilled typist, for instance, should perform her task with less energy expenditure than a novice as she would be economical with her movements. A trained bricklayer would pace himself better over a day's work than an untrained man, and an athlete running would expend less energy than an untrained man running the same distance. But the figures do provide a reasonable estimate of the energy expended in the activities shown.

Modern day man and woman, especially in cities and towns, are less active than their ancestors and their energy needs are, therefore, lower. It is customary to divide the town dweller's day into three parts, each with its own energy needs: eight hours spent in bed or asleep, eight hours spent at work, and eight hours for leisure activities like gardening, sports, or watching television.

The daily round

Here is the level of energy expended by a young married couple during the course of a typical weekday. Mr Reid is 30 and is a junior public relations consultant.

Mrs Reid, who is 28, is essentially a housewife, but also does some typing at home.

Mr Reid

		Calories
11.30 pm to 7.30 am	Asleep in bed	500
7.30 am to 8.30 am	Getting up, and breakfast	210
8.30 am to 9.30 am	Briskly walking to the office	300
9.30 am to 5.30 pm	Mostly sitting down in the office	850
5.30 pm to 6.30 pm	Public transport home	120
6.30 pm to 7.30 pm	Bathing and dressing for dinner	180
7.30 pm to 8.30 pm	Dinner	80
8.30 pm to 11.30 pm	Watching TV	250
Total calorie expenditure		**2490**

Mrs Reid

		Calories
11.30 pm to 7.30 am	Asleep in bed	420
7.30 am to 8.30 am	Getting up and preparing breakfast	200
8.30 am to 9.30 am	Housework	150
9.30 am to 1.30 pm	Typing at home	130
1.30 pm to 2.30 pm	Lunch, read newspaper	60
2.30 pm to 4.30 pm	Typing	65
4.30 pm to 5.00 pm	Walking to club	90
5.00 pm to 6.30 pm	Tennis	450
6.30 pm to 7.30 pm	Shower, dress and walk home	210
7.30 pm to 8.30 pm	Dinner, almost no cooking	65
8.30 pm to 11.30 pm	Watching TV	216
Total calorie expenditure		**2056**

Mr and Mrs Reid's day is rather a sedentary one. In spite of Mrs Reid's walk to and from the club and the hour and a half of tennis, and although it is not easy to be accurate in assessing how much energy an individual expends, both would fit easily into the group who need rather a low daily intake of food. This does not mean, of course, that they are not getting enough to eat. They are an example of how hard it is to label anyone as *average*. At work, Mr Reid seems to spend much of his time at his desk; not one of those PR men who rush about. Within the ranks of men or women in any occupation, the actual work done in terms of energy varies from person to person. In heavy work, like sawing wood, a man may not be at it all day and every hour, and may if he is lazy, expend less energy than a man who is hard at work all day as a carpenter.

Fitting Yourself into a group
Most women are thought to need 880 Calories whether at home, in the office, or the factory, with another 900 Calories for work or play plus 420 Calories for time spent in bed. Very active women can

Your lifestyle will dictate your energy expenditure group.

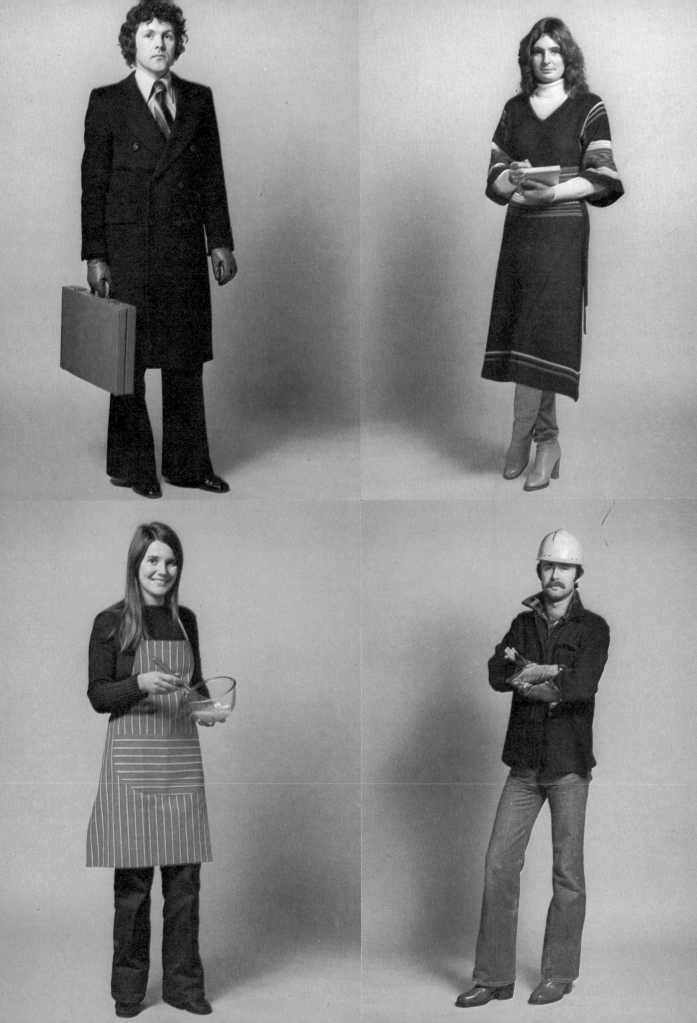

allow themselves another 300 Calories a day.
Recommended Calorie intake: 2200 Calories or 2500 Calories a day.

Most men can put themselves into one of these three groups, each with its recommended Calorie intake.

The sedentary group includes doctors, lawyers, architects, journalists, teachers, shop assistants, office workers, and drivers.
Recommended Calorie intake: 2700 a day.

The moderately active group includes the postman, the plumber, the bus conductor, the carpenter, the railwayman, some farm workers, some labourers in the building trade, unskilled labourers, and anyone in light industry or on assembly plant.
Recommended Calorie intake: 3000 Calories a day.

The very active group includes some farm workers, builders' labourers, coal miners, dockers, forestry workers, army recruits.
Recommended Calorie intake: 3600 Calories a day.

What difference do hobbies make?
Hobbies, whether very active ones like some sports, moderate like gardening, or light like golf, affect the daily Calorie expenditure of an individual. But there is no evidence that your occupational group at work matches what you do in your spare time. Plenty of office workers have been very active amateur boxers, for instance, and it is not unknown for a factory worker to spend a lot of spare time reading or watching television.

Special Groups of People
These are the young, the old, and the pregnant. Recommended Calorie intake for the young is as follows:

Boys and Girls

Up to 1 year	800 Calories
1 to 2 years	1200 Calories
2 to 3 years	1400 Calories
3 to 5 years	1600 Calories
5 to 7 years	1800 Calories
7 to 9 years	2100 Calories

A woman can burn up to 6 Calories per minute cycling.

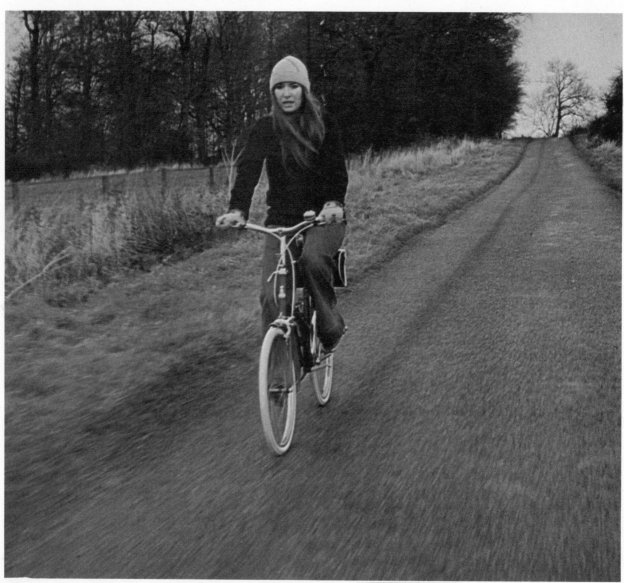

Boys

9 to 12 years	2500 Calories
12 to 15 years	2800 Calories
15 to 18 years	3000 Calories

Girls

9 to 12 years	2300 Calories
12 to 15 years	2300 Calories
15 to 18 years	2300 Calories

The reason the recommended intake is unaltered for girls is because obesity is so common among this age group that they should be encouraged to eat less, though keeping to a balanced diet.

The elderly

Age brings a lower basic rate of metabolism, and, in most people, a slowing down in activity. There are exceptions, of course, and some people, as is common knowledge, remain extremely active in their seventies and eighties, and will need more than the recommended amounts.
Recommended Calorie intakes are:

Men

65 to 75 years and sedentary	2350 Calories
75 and over and sedentary	2100 Calories

Women

55 to 75 years and sedentary	2050 Calories
75 and over and sedentary	1900 Calories

Pregnant women

A mother has to provide all the energy and nutrients for the growing baby in her womb. Extra food is laid down as fat to be drawn on later when the mother is secreting milk but, since pregnancy is one of the triggers of later obesity, doctors usually advise mothers not to eat more than they need at this time.
Recommended Calorie intake during last six months of pregnancy: 2400
Recommended Calorie intake when breast feeding: 2700

Energy used in some common activities

The figures given here are for the amount of Calories used per minute by the average man and woman.

	Average man Calories	Average woman Calories
Sitting watching TV	1.4	1.2
In bed asleep	1.1	0.9
Looking out of the window	1.8	1.4
Cooking	2.1	1.7
Dusting	3.1	2.5
Scrubbing	4.3	3.5
In the office	1.8	1.6
Driving a car	1.6	1.4
Walking easily	3.7	3.0
Walking briskly	5.0	4.0
Dancing	5 to 7.5	4 to 6
Gardening	5 to 7.4	4 to 6
Bicycling	5 to 7.4	4 to 6

Energy value of some everyday food and drink

The Calorie content given for the following selection of everyday foods is expressed in amounts per 28g [1oz], together with a comparison in relation to this amount or the amount generally served as a typical helping. To find the Calorie content for a typical helping multiply the Calories by the amount of food.

	Calories	Typical Helping
White bread	72	28g is 1 slice
Wholemeal bread	68	28g is 1 slice
Crispbread	90	28g is 3 crispbreads
Cornflakes	100	28g
Rice	102	113g [4oz] boiled
Pasta	103	113g [4oz] cooked
Bacon	126	28g is 1 slice
Corned beef	61	28g is 1½ slices
Roast beef	64	28g is ½ slice
Roast chicken	42	28g is ½ slice
Roast lamb	83	28g is ½ slice
Roast pork	94	28g is ½ slice
Pork sausage	104	28g is ½ sausage
Beef sausage	84	28g is ½ sausage
Steak and kidney pie	86	170g [6oz]
Fried liver	70	113g [4oz]
Ham	77	28g [1oz] is 1 thin slice
Fish fingers [sticks]	51	28g [1oz] is 1 finger
Kipper	52	113g [4oz]
Herring	66	113g [4oz]
Canned sardines	84	85g [3oz]
Cod, haddock and white fish	23	113g [4oz]
Egg	42	28g is ½ egg
Cheddar cheese	117	56g [2oz]
Cottage cheese	32	113g [4oz]
Butter	207	8g [¼oz] per slice
Margarine	208	8g [¼oz] per slice
Oil	255	28g
Dripping	254	28g
Milk	19	285ml [10oz]
Double [thick] cream	127	28g is 2 tablespoons
Yoghurt	15	140g [5oz]
Marmalade	74	14g [½oz]
White sugar	112	28g is 1 tablespoon
Baked beans in tomato sauce	17	113g [4oz]
Brussel sprouts	5	113g [4oz]
Lettuce	2	14g [½oz]
Carrots	6	113g [4oz]
Boiled potatoes	23	113g [4oz] is 1 large
Chips	68	85g [3oz]
Spinach	7	113g [4oz]
Apple	13	113g [4oz] is 1 apple
Banana	22	85g [3oz] is 1 banana
Dates	70	113g [4oz] is 10 dates
Orange	10	113g [4oz] is 1 orange
Cucumber	3	28g is 5 slices
Beer	9	570ml [20oz]
Gin and whisky	62	standard measure 24ml
Dry wine	21	110ml [4oz]
Sweet wine	24	110ml [4oz]
Ice cream	55	56g [2oz]

DESIGNED FOR YOU

Using the nutrition chart you can plan a slimming diet to suit yourself. Once you have lost enough weight to bring you to your ideal weight, you can use the chart to plan your daily meals.

Remember always that a slimming diet is one that cuts down your energy intake while still providing the protein, minerals and vitamins you must have to maintain a healthy body. A slimming diet is still a balanced diet.

All slimming diets are 'low calorie' diets. The aim is always to keep the energy intake below your daily energy needs so that the extra energy comes from the body's fat stores.

Choosing a diet for yourself is a matter of personal choice. It is important to be in good health before you start on a weight reducing diet and you would be wise to consult your doctor before you attempt any drastic reducing.

A reasonable daily cut back is 1000 Calories, which will give an approximate loss of 7000 Calories a week, the energy equivalent of one kilo [2 pounds] of fat.

Looking at the nutrition chart you will see that most foods contain several nutrients and that everyday foods contain enough minerals, vitamins and protein for a balanced diet.

It follows that the simplest way to ensure a balanced diet is to choose from a wide range of everyday foods. One reason why some slimming diets are unsuitable is that they ignore this fact and by concentrating on grapefruit or yoghurt or bananas or some other food, provide a boring and unhealthy diet which is hard to

stick to and does not re-educate your eating habits.

Remember, the best pattern for a slimmer should be three or four small meals daily. This speeds up metabolism more than one or two larger meals a day. The content of these meals should include reasonable amounts of the high quality protein foods such as meat, fish, cheese or eggs, plenty of fruit and vegetables, but not very much bread or potato.

With these basic principles in mind it is time to look at the three most practical diet plans and choose the one that would best suit you. For instance, it is unwise to follow the Calorie counting plan if counting and simple arithmetic bore you. Nor is the low carbohydrate plan suitable if you have a sweet tooth or like a drink—too difficult to resist temptation.

Calorie counting plan

Following this plan entails checking the Calorie content of *everything* you eat and drink and ensuring that the total consumed adds up to the number you have allotted yourself. It is low in energy intake but still a balanced diet.

When you have been on the Calorie counting diet for a few days you will find that the counting becomes easier because you won't have to consult the chart so much: the Calorie content of the food and drink you turn to most often becomes easy to remember.

Counting Calories does not mean starving yourself—the meal of pie and chips, pastry and beer contains more Calories than the wide selection of food in the other meal.

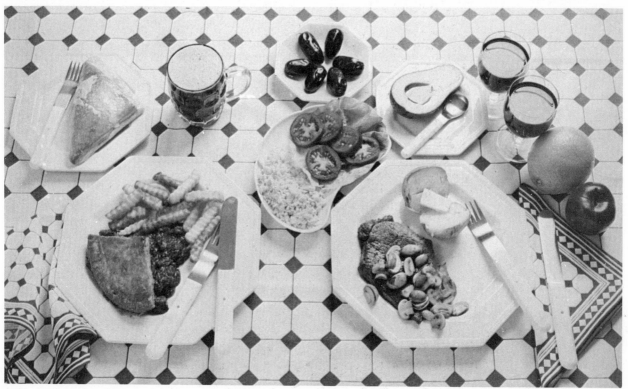

Low carbohydrate plan

Some arithmetic needed but not much. The great advantage of this plan is that by cutting down on carbohydrate-rich food and drink you will find yourself eating less fat as well (less bread means less butter or margarine on it), and you will be eating more of the nutrient-rich food because you are avoiding the food that provides 'empty calories' (just energy and no nutrients).

The aim should be no more than 50 grams of carbohydrate a day. The chart shows the number of carbohydrate grams contained in 28 grams [one ounce] of each food.

The drawback to the low carbohydrate plan is the temptation to eat too much of non-carbohydrate containing food in the mistaken belief that the Calories, the energy content, in meat, fish, cheese and eggs do not matter. They do. All these foods have an energy content and the slimmer still needs to stick to a low energy diet. The choice lies in the method of doing so.

No-count plan

With this plan you do not count calories but avoid certain foods altogether, eat as much as you like of others and a little of a few more.
Avoid all kinds of bread, including brown bread and starch-reduced bread. Anything made with flour, such as white sauce, thick soup, gravy, cakes, pies, pastry, biscuits or cookies, puddings, pasta, breakfast cereals. All sugar, sweets, chocolate, sweet drinks, jam, honey, marmalade, syrup, treacle, canned fruit, nuts, cocktail titbits, potatoes, rice, bananas and ALCOHOL.
Have plenty of meat, poultry, fish, game, eggs, offal [organ meats], green vegetables, fruit, unsweetened tea or coffee, water.
Have some of butter, margarine, cheese, 285ml [half pint] milk daily, root vegetables, peas and beans, cream, fats and oils.

The drawback to this plan is that again you might be tempted to eat too much of the foods you are allowed plenty of because they are low in carbohydrate or relatively so. Cost of food will be a little more because you are eating high-protein food rather than high carbohydrate food and it is generally more expensive.

Putting the diet into practice

After looking at the ideal weight chart and remembering what she used to weigh at the time of her marriage, Mrs Reid, who we met earlier, has decided that she is six kilos [14 pounds] overweight. She knows that she eats too much and takes too little exercise. In other words, she is losing her figure and is alarmed by it. She opts for the Calorie counting plan, with the addition of a daily stint of exercises to improve her waistline. Sensibly, she aims to lose 1000 Calories a day by sticking to a 1500 Calorie per day diet for seven weeks. She hopes to lose 7000 Calories, the equivalent of one kilo [two pounds] a week by doing this. She looks on the extra Calories used up by the daily exercises as a bonus—chiefly to improve her posture and tighten her muscles.

Working out a menu

Mrs Reid draws up a list, meal by meal, of her favourite and standard food. Luckily her husband has the same tastes, so she does not have to worry about pleasing him separately.

Turning to the chart, she then put against each item chosen for the day's menu, its Calorie content and its protein content, if any. With some juggling, cutting out here and adding there, she provided a 1500 Calorie menu. Turning then to the chart showing the recommended daily intake of nutrients, she was delighted to find that she had a little more than the daily recommendation of protein. She also made sure, quite rightly, that the foods chosen would be providing enough minerals and vitamins.

A typical day's menu

		Calories	Protein (grams)
Breakfast	½ large grapefruit	15	0.5
	Boiled egg	80	6.8
	2 large slices of wholemeal bread	140	4.6
Mid-morning	Cup of tea or coffee with milk	20	0.9
Lunch	Slice of melon (Cantaloupe)	16	0.6
	170g [6oz] plaice fillet	126	29.4
	Large helping of cabbage	30	3.0
	1 boiled potato	92	1.6
	1 orange	40	0.8
Mid-afternoon	Cup of tea or coffee with milk	20	0.9
Evening	113g [4oz] roast chicken	168	28
	1 baked potato	92	1.6
	113g [4oz] carrots	24	0.8
	56g [2oz] cottage cheese	64	8.6
	2 plain crackers (table water)	126	3.0
	28g [1oz] butter	207	0.1
Nightcap	425ml [¾ pint] hot milk	300	14.4
	Total	**1560**	**105.6**

Using the charts, the daily menu can be varied according to taste. Once Mrs Reid has reached her ideal weight, she resolves to be careful to increase her energy intake slowly and not to rush back to her old eating habits. She decides to replace 200 Calories a week until she reaches the recommended intake for a person of her age and occupation—that is, 2200 Calories. And she will never give up her daily dozen!

BALANCED OUT
NUTRITION CHART

The nutrition chart has been specially prepared to help you to evaluate the foods you wish to include in your meals—not only for slimming but also for planning the weekly shopping list and menus.

The chart includes a wide variety of foods which have been given in measurements of 28g [1oz] for easy Calorie counting. For instance, 28g [1oz] of grilled beef steak contains 86 Calories, so a 170g [6oz] steak would give you 516 Calories, plus a quantity of protein and fat. (Vitamins and minerals are included only when the food is a 'reliable' source of them.)

You will be surprised at how quickly you learn how to evaluate and understand the nutritional value of the foods you buy—you might even find yourself trying out foods that you wouldn't previously have thought of buying!

The chart has been divided into sections for easy reference.

Meat
Meat is an excellent source of high quality protein which does not have to come from the most expensive cuts. 113 grams [four ounces] of rump steak will provide the same quality 20 grams of protein as 113 grams [four ounces] of *lean* meat from stewing steak. Although meat is valued chiefly for its protein, water outweighs the protein. The fat content varies from cut to cut of meat as well as from different types of meat.

Chicken meat and offal [organ meats] are lower in calories because they have less fat.

Fish
Fish is also an excellent source of high quality protein.

White fish, like cod or haddock, have less fat than the oily fish like herring, salmon, mackerel, trout and eel and their flesh does not carry the fat-soluble vitamins A and D as these do. High protein and low energy content make fish ideal for a slimming diet.

Salt-water fish and shell-fish are a good source of iodine and canned fish such as tuna, salmon, sardine, are rich in phosphorus and calcium.

Vegetables
Many vegetables can be a very useful part of the slimmer's diet because of their 'filling' qualities and low energy content. They contain 80 to 90 per cent water but also many nutrients; they are often fat-free and low in carbohydrates.

Pulses or legumes like peas, beans and other seeds like lentils are better sources of protein and energy than other vegetables. They often form the basis of a balanced vegetarian diet.

All vegetables contain fibre which is largely indigestible and so adds bulk to the diet.

Potatoes are the chief source in many people's diets of vitamin C. Less vitamin C is lost in cooking potatoes than in cooking some other common vegetables.

Fruit
Fruit, fresh not dried, is low in energy and therefore an important substitute for puddings in slimming diets. Bananas and grapes are exceptions since they contain quite a lot of sugar. Dried fruit like figs, dates, and prunes contain much less water than fresh fruit and so are even higher in energy, weight for weight.

Fresh fruit is most important as a source of vitamin C. In Western countries it supplies about one third of the total need. Blackcurrants and rosehips are richest in vitamin C. Strawberries, oranges, grapefruit, and lemons contain fair amounts, but apples and cherries have less.

Nuts
Nuts are rich sources of protein, fat, fibre and some of the B vitamins. Chestnuts, however, contain much carbohydrate and little protein and fat.

Peanuts have most protein, followed by Brazil nuts and walnuts, all as good a source of protein as eggs or cheese.

Dairy produce
Milk is the most comprehensive in nutrients of all foods but because of its high energy content needs to be treated with care by slimmers. A pint of milk has the same energy value as four large slices of bread.

Butter is concentrated milk fat and therefore very high in energy value and to be eaten sparingly in a low calorie diet. A rich source of vitamin A, some D and E.

Cheese is almost carbohydrate-free and high in fat and protein, therefore a good source of energy. Cheddar cheese is one third fat, one third protein and one third water. It is only the cottage cheese and curd cheese which are usually made from skimmed milk that are good for slimming diets as they contain little fat.

Eggs contain practically no carbohydrate and no vitamin C but they are a good source of all other nutrients. The yolk, weighing one third of the egg, is the main source. It contains 16 per cent protein, 30 per cent fat, vitamins A, B, D, E, calcium, iron and other minerals.

Cereals
'Give us this day our daily bread' must not be taken literally by slimmers because, unlike the rest of the world, they should not rely so much on cereals as a

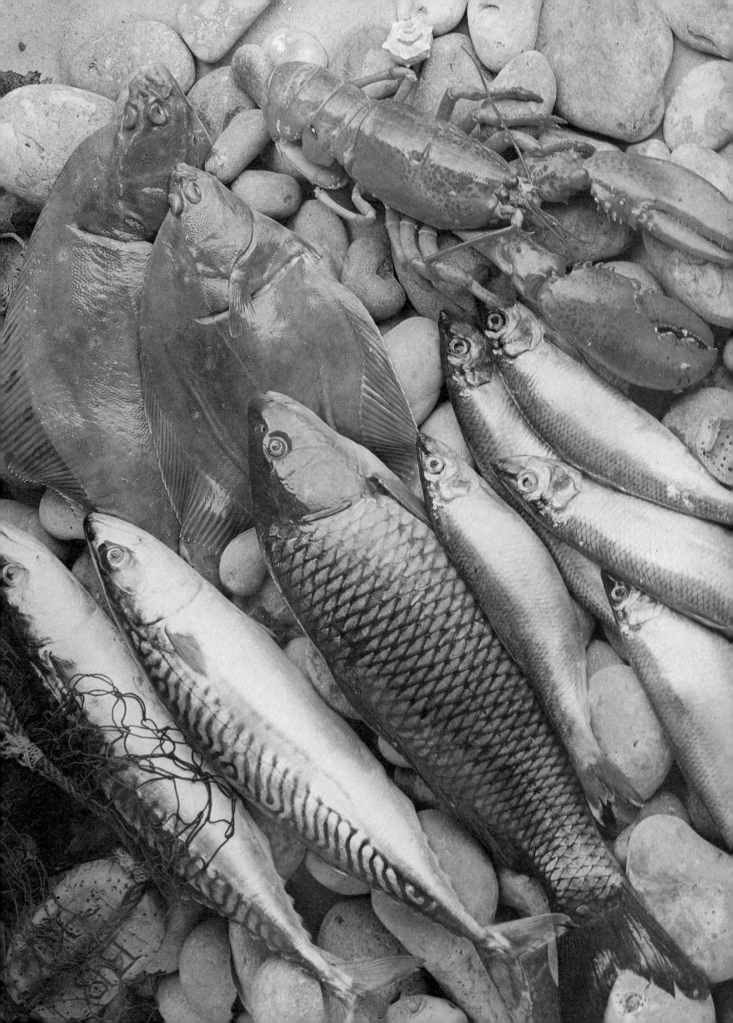

major food. In an average Western family, the wheat in bread, cakes, flour, pasta and biscuits, crackers and cookies, plus other cereals provide between a quarter and a third of all the energy, protein, carbohydrate and iron in the diet.

Biscuits and cookies; Puddings, pastries and cakes; Sugars, sweets and candies; Condiments

Nutritionally, none of these foods is a necessary part of the diet. White sugar is a source of energy only. Brown sugar contains tiny amounts of minerals and B vitamins, but nothing like enough to be important.

About half the sugar eaten in the Western world is consumed via cooking and in sweetening tea and coffee.

For slimmers, all these foods are superfluous and can be left out of the diet without risk to health.

Liquids

A daily intake of at least 568 ml or one pint of water is essential. Ordinary drinking water contains calcium, magnesium and other salts.

Fruit squash, fruit cordial, fruit drinks whether sparkling or still have, as their main ingredients, water and sugar.

Alcohol has an energy value of seven Calories a gram, almost as much as fat. Since alcohol is used for energy before carbohydrate and fat are called on, the constant drinker tends to put on weight.

FOOD	Calories	Protein g	Fat g	Carbohy-drate g	Reliable Mineral Source	Reliable Vitamin Source
Meat			Composition per 28g [1 oz] raw edible weight unless stated otherwise			
Bacon back [salt pork], fried	169	7.0	15.2	0	Iron, Phosphorus	B
Bacon [Canadian], crispy	149	6.8	13.1	0	Iron, Phosphorus	B
Bacon, gammon, fried	126	8.9	9.6	0	Iron, Phosphorus	B
Beef, corned	61	7.6	3.4	0	Iron, Phosphorus	A, B
Beef, mince [ground], grilled	55	7	7	0	Iron, Phosphorus	B
Beef, lean and fat, roast	109	6.0	9.1	0	Iron, Phosphorus	B
Beef, lean sirloin, roast	64	7.6	3.5	0	Iron, Phosphorus	B
Beef, silverside	86	7.9	5.7	0	Iron, Phosphorus	B
Beef steak, fried	78	5.8	5.8	0	Iron, Phosphorus	B
Beef steak, grilled	86	7.2	6.1	0	Iron, Phosphorus	B
Beef, steak and kidney pie	86	3.8	6.0	4.6	Iron, Phosphorus	A, B
Beef steak, raw	50	5.5	3.0	0	Iron, Phosphorus	A, B
Beef steak, stewed	58	8.7	2.4	0	Iron, Phosphorus	B
Black [blood] pudding	87	3.7	6.2	4.3	Iron, Phosphorus	B
Brains (calf)	29	3.4	1.6	0	Iron, Phosphorus	A, B
Chicken, boiled	28	6.9	2.1	0	Iron, Phosphorus	B
Chicken, fried	35	7.1	3.1	0	Iron, Phosphorus	B
Chicken, fried in egg and breadcrumbs	42	7.9	4.3	3	Iron, Phosphorus	B
Chicken, roast	42	7.0	1.5	0	Iron, Phosphorus	B
Duck, roast	89	6.5	6.7	0	Iron, Phosphorus	B
Goose, roast	92	8.0	6.4	0		

FOOD	Calories	Protein g	Fat g	Carbohydrate g	Reliable Mineral Source	Reliable Vitamin Source
Grouse	49	8.6	1.5	0		
Guinea fowl, roast	60	9.2	2.3	0		
Ham	77	7.0	5.4	0	Iron, Phosphorus	B
Hamburger with cereal	70	7	7	2	Iron, Phosphorus	B
Hare, stewed	55	8.3	2.3	0	Iron, Phosphorus	B
Heart (sheep's), roasted	68	7.1	4.2	0	Iron, Phosphorus	B
Kidney	26	4.6	0.8	0	Iron, Phosphorus	A, B
Lamb, chops, grilled	36	3.5	2.3	0	Iron, Phosphorus	B
Lamb, roast	83	6.5	6.3	0	Iron, Phosphorus	B
Liver, fried	70	7.1	3.9	1.6	Iron, Phosphorus	A, B
Luncheon meat	89	3.6	7.6	1.6	Phosphorus	B
Meat paste	61	5.6	3.6	1.2	Iron, Phosphorus	B
Partridge, roast	60	10	2	0	Iron, Phosphorus	B
Pheasant, roast	61	8.8	2.6	0	Iron, Phosphorus	B
Pigeon, roast	66	7.6	3.8	0	Iron, Phosphorus	B
Pork chop, grilled	94	8.1	6.9	0	Phosphorus	B
Pork, roast	94	4.5	8.4	0	Phosphorus	B
Rabbit, stewed	26	3.9	1.1	0	Phosphorus	B
Sausage, beef	84	2.7	6.8	3.3	Iron, Phosphorus	B
Sausage, pork	104	3.0	9.1	2.7	Iron, Phosphorus	B
Sweetbreads, stewed	51	6.4	2.6	0	Iron, Phosphorus	B
Tongue (ox)	88	5.4	6.8	0.7	Iron, Phosphorus	B
Tripe	72	2.7	0.7	0	Calcium	A, B
Turkey, roast	56	8.6	2.2	0	Iron, Phosphorus	B
Veal chop, grilled	70	7.8	3	0	Iron, Phosphorus	B
Veal fillet, roast	56	9.5	3.3	0	Iron, Phosphorus	B
Venison, roast	56	9.5	1.8	0	Iron, Phosphorus	B

Fish

FOOD	Calories	Protein g	Fat g	Carbohydrate g	Reliable Mineral Source	Reliable Vitamin Source
Abalone, canned	23	3.3	0.5	0.6	Phosphorus	A , B
Anchovy	50	5.8	2.1	0	Phosphorus, Iodine	A, D, E, B
Bass, steamed	36	5.5	1.5	0	Phosphorus, Iodine	B

FOOD	Calories	Protein g	Fat g	Carbohy-drate g	Reliable Mineral Source	Reliable Vitamin Source
Bloaters [Cisco], grilled	73	6.4	4.9	0	Phosphorus, Iodine	A, D
Bream, steamed	34	5.6	1.1	0	Phosphorus, Iodine	B
Brill	33	5.8	1.0	0	Phosphorus, Iodine	B
Carp	32	6.2	1.1	0	Phosphorus	B
Catfish, steamed	34	5.8	1.1	0	Phosphorus, Iodine	B
Caviar (sturgeon)	62	6.8	4.0	0	Phosphorus	B
Clams	23	3.3	0.4	1.7	Phosphorus, Calcium, Iodine	B
Cockles	14	3.1	0.1	Tr	Phosphorus, Iodine, Iron	B
Cod, fried in batter	56	5.6	2.9	2.1	Phosphorus, Iodine	B
Cod, grilled	45	7.7	1.5	0	Phosphorus, Iodine	B
Cod, steamed	23	5.1	0.3	0	Phosphorus, Iodine	B
Cod roe, fried	59	5.8	3.4	0.9	Phosphorus, Iodine, Iron	B
Conger eel, steamed	23	4.9	0.4	0	Phosphorus, Iodine	B
Crab, boiled	36	5.4	1.5	0	Phosphorus, Calcium, Iron	B
Dabs, fried	71	5.5	4.1	2.8	Phosphorus, Iodine	B
Eels, jellied	110	5.0	9.2	0	Phosphorus, Iodine	A, B, D
Eels, stewed	106	5.0	9.2	0	Phosphorus, Iodine	A, B, D
Fish fingers [sticks]	51	3.6	2.1	4.6	Phosphorus, Iodine	B
Fish paste	49	4.2	2.7	1.9	Phosphorus	B
Flounder	22	3.8	0.2	0	Phosphorus Iodine	B
Haddock, fried, dipped in egg with breadcrumbs	46	6.2	4	1.8	Phosphorus, Iodine	B
Haddock, smoked	28	6.3	0.3	0	Phosphorus, Iodine	B
Haddock, steamed	28	6.2	0.2	0	Phosphorus, Iodine	B

FOOD	Calories	Protein g	Fat g	Carbohy-drate g	Reliable Mineral Source	Reliable Vitamin Source
Hake, fried	58	5.5	3.2	1.5	Phosphorus, Iodine	B
Halibut, fried	49	6.5	7.3	0	Phosphorus, Iodine	B
Halibut, steamed	37	6.4	1.1	0	Phosphorus, Iodine	B
Herring	66	4.8	5.2	0	Phosphorus, Calcium, Iodine, Iron	A, D, B
Herring, pickled	62	4.5	3.2	0	Phosphorus, Iodine, Calcium, Iron	A, D, B
Herring, smoked	55	4.5	3.2	0	Phosphorus, Iodine	A, D, B
Kipper	52	5.6	3.3	0	Phosphorus, Iodine	A, D, B
Lobster, boiled	34	6.0	1.0	0	Phosphorus, Calcium, Iodine, Iron	B
Mackerel, canned	52	5.0	3.1	0	Phosphorus, Iodine	A, D, B
Mackerel, smoked	28	6.0	0.2	0	Phosphorus, Iodine	A, D, B
Mussels, boiled	25	4.4	0.6	Tr	Phosphorus, Calcium, Iodine, Iron	B
Octopus	21	3.3	0.4	0	Phosphorus	B
Oysters	14	2.9	0.3	Tr	Phosphorus, Calcium, Iodine, Iron	B
Perch	33	6.3	1.1	0	Phosphorus	B
Pilchards, canned inc. juice	63	5.4	4.4	0	Phosphorus, Iodine, Calcium	B, A, D
Plaice, fried	66	5.1	4.1	2.0	Phosphorus, Iodine	B
Plaice, steamed	26	5.1	0.5	0	Phosphorus, Iodine	B
Prawns	30	6.0	0.5	0	Phosphorus, Iron, Calcium, Iodine	B
Red mullet, steamed	36	6.1	1.2	0	Phosphorus, Iodine	A, D, B
Salmon, canned	39	5.6	1.7	0	Phosphorus, Iodine	A, D, B
Salmon, grilled	57	5.4	3.7	0	Phosphorus, Iodine	A, D, B

FOOD	Calories	Protein g	Fat g	Carbohy-drate g	Reliable Mineral Source	Reliable Vitamin Source
Salmon, smoked	48	5.4	3.7	0	Phosphorus, Iodine	A, D, B
Sardines, canned	84	5.8	6.4	0	Phosphorus, Calcium, Iodine, Iron	A, B, D
Scallops, steamed	30	6.4	0.4	Tr	Phosphorus, Calcium, Iodine, Iron	B
Shrimps	32	6.3	0.7	0	Phosphorus, Calcium, Iodine, Iron	B
Skate, fried	69	4.3	4.7	2.1	Phosphorus, Iodine	B
Sole, Lemon, fried	62	4.4	3.7	2.6	Phosphorus, Iodine	B
Sole, Lemon, steamed	24	5	0.4	0	Phosphorus, Iodine	B
Sprats, fried	126	6.3	10.8	0	Phosphorus, Calcium, Iodine, Iron	B
Sturgeon, steamed	44	7.0	1.6	0	Phosphorus	B
Trout, steamed	37	6.0	1.4	0	Phosphorus, Iodine	B
Tuna, canned in oil	80	6.0	6.1	0	Phosphorus, Iodine, Iron	A, B, D
Turbot, steamed	28	5.9	0.5	0	Phosphorus, Iodine	B
Whelks	26	5.1	0.5	Tr	Phosphorus, Iodine, Iron	B
Whitebait, fried	152	5.2	13.5	1.5	Phosphorus, Iodine, Calcium,	B
Whiting, fried	55	4.9	2.9	2.0	Phosphorus, Iodine	B
Winkles [Periwinkles] boiled in fresh water	4	0.7	0.1	Tr	Phosphorus, Iodine, Iron	B

Vegetables

FOOD	Calories	Protein g	Fat g	Carbohy-drate g	Reliable Mineral Source	Reliable Vitamin Source
Artichokes, globe, boiled	4	0.3	Tr	0.8	Calcium, Magnesium	C, B
Artichokes, Jerusalem, boiled	5	0.1	Tr	0.9	Calcium, Iron, Potassium	C, B, A
Asparagus, boiled	5	1.0	Tr	0.3	Calcium, Iron, Potassium	C, B, A
Aubergine [egg plant], raw	4	0.2	Tr	0.9	Potassium	

FOOD	Calories	Protein g	Fat g	Carbohy-drate g	Reliable Mineral Source	Reliable Vitamin Source
Aubergine [egg plant], baked	4	0.2	Tr	0.9	Potassium	
Bamboo shoots, raw	8	0.2	0	5.9	Potassium	
Bamboo shoots, boiled	7	0.2	0	5.9	Potassium	
Beans, baked	26	1.8	0.1	4.9	Potassium	B
Beans, broad, boiled	12	1.2	Tr	2.0	Potassium	B, C
Beans, butter, boiled	26	2.0	Tr	4.9	Potassium	B
Beans, French, boiled	2	0.2	Tr	0.3	Potassium	C
Beans, haricot, boiled	25	1.9	Tr	4.7	Calcium, Phosphorus, Potassium	B, C
Beans, runner, boiled	2	0.2	Tr	0.3	Potassium	B
Beetroot [beets], boiled	13	0.5	Tr	2.8	Potassium	
Broccoli, boiled	4	0.9	Tr	0.1	Calcium, Potassium	C
Brussels sprouts, boiled	5	0.7	Tr	0.5	Potassium	A, C, B
Cabbage, boiled, green	5	0.5	0	0.7	Potassium	C, B, A
Cabbage, red, raw	6	0.5	Tr	1.0	Potassium	C
Cabbage, Chinese	4	0.8	0	1.05	Potassium	C
Carrots, boiled, old	5	0.2	Tr	1.2	Potassium	A
Carrots, canned	5	0.2	Tr	1.2	Potassium	A
Carrots, raw, old	6	0.2	Tr	1.5	Potassium	A
Carrots, young, boiled	6	0.3	Tr	1.3	Potassium	A
Cauliflower, boiled	3	0.4	Tr	0.3	Iron, Potassium	B
Celery, boiled	1	0.2	Tr	0.2	Potassium	B
Celery, raw	3	0.3	Tr	0.4	Potassium	B
Chickpeas	76	2.3	Tr	6.2	Potassium	B
Chicory, raw	3	0.2	Tr	0.4	Potassium	
Coleslaw with mayonnaise	130	0.3	15	1.2	Potassium	C
Courgette [zucchini]	17	0.1	0.9	2.1	Potassium	
Cucumber, raw	3	0.2	Tr	0.5	Potassium	
Endive, raw	3	0.5	Tr	0.3	Potassium	
Horseradish, raw	17	1.3	Tr	3.1	Calcium, Potassium	
Kale, boiled	11	0.9	Tr	1.7	Potassium	
Leeks, boiled	7	0.5	Tr	1.3	Potassium	B

FOOD	Calories	Protein g	Fat g	Carbohy- drate g	Reliable Mineral Source	Reliable Vitamin Source
Lentils, boiled	27	1.9	Tr	5.2	Iron, Potassium	B
Lettuce, raw	3	0.3	Tr	0.5	Potassium	A, B, C
Marrow, boiled	2	0.1	Tr	0.4	Potassium	
Mushrooms, raw	2	0.5	Tr	0	Phosphorus, Potassium	B
Mushrooms, sauteed	62	0.6	6.4	0	Potassium	B
Mustard and cress	3	0.5	Tr	0.3	Calcium, Iron, Potassium	C
Okra, boiled	9	0.5	Tr	1.7	Potassium	
Onions, boiled	4	0.2	Tr	0.8	Potassium	B, C
Onions, fried	101	0.5	9.5	2.9	Potassium	B, C
Onions, raw	7	0.3	Tr	1.5	Potassium	B, C
Onions, spring, raw	10	0.3	Tr	2.4	Potassium	B, C
Parsley, raw	6	1.5	Tr	Tr	Iron, Potassium	C
Parsnips, baked	16	0.4	Tr	3.8	Iron Potassium,	B
Parsnips, boiled	15	0.4	Tr	3.8	Iron, Potassium	C
Peas, canned	24	1.7	Tr	4.7	Potassium	
Peas, dried, boiled	28	2.0	Tr	5.4	Potassium	B
Peas, fresh, boiled	14	1.4	Tr	2.2	Potassium	C, B
Peas, split, dried, boiled	33	2.3	Tr	6.2	Potassium	B
Peas, frozen	18	1.6	Tr	3.0	Potassium	C, B
Peppers, cooked	5	0.3	Tr	1.7	Potassium	C
Peppers, raw	7	0.3	Tr	1.7	Potassium	C
Potatoes, baked	24	0.6	Tr	5.8	Potassium	C, B
Potatoes, boiled, new	21	0.5	Tr	5.2	Potassium	C, B
Potatoes, boiled, old	23	0.4	Tr	5.6	Potassium	C, B
Potatoes, canned	25	0.4	Tr	5.6	Potassium	B, C (if added)
Potatoes, old, chips [French fried]	68	1.1	2.6	10.6	Potassium	C, B, E
Potato crisps [chips]	159	1.7	10.2	14.0	Potassium	C, B, E
Potatoes, dried plus milk	35	0.4	1.4	5.2	Potassium	B, C (if added)
Potatoes, old, mashed with milk and butter	34	0.4	1.4	5.1	Potassium	C, B, E
Potatoes, roast, old	35	0.8	0.3	7.8	Potassium	C, B, E
Potato salad	32	1.8	5.4	5	Potassium	C, B, E

FOOD	Calories	Protein g	Fat g	Carbohy-drate g	Reliable Mineral Source	Reliable Vitamin Source
Pumpkin, boiled	4	0.2	Tr	1.0	Potassium	
Radishes	4	0.3	Tr	0.8	Potassium	
Spinach, boiled	7	1.4	Tr	0.4	Calcium, Iron, Potassium	B, A, K, C
Spring greens, boiled	3	0.5	Tr	0.3	Potassium	C, B
Squash (winter), boiled	12	0.4	Tr	3.0	Potassium	
Swedes [rutabagas], boiled	23	0.3	Tr	1.1	Potassium	C
Sweetcorn, boiled	24	1.3	0.1	4.2	Potassium	A, B, E
Sweetcorn, canned	26	0.5	0.1	5.2	Potassium	A, B, E
Sweet potatoes, boiled	23	0.3	Tr	5.7	Potassium	A
Tomatoes, fried	20	0.3	1.7	0.9	Potassium	A, C
Tomatoes, raw	4	0.3	Tr	0.8	Potassium	A, C
Turnips, boiled	3	0.2	Tr	0.7	Poatssium	C
Watercress	4	0.8	Tr	0.2	Calcium, Potassium	A, B, C
Yam, boiled	32	0.4	Tr	7.7	Potassium	

Fruit

FOOD	Calories	Protein g	Fat g	Carbohy-drate g	Reliable Mineral Source	Reliable Vitamin Source
Apple	13	0.1	0	3.4		
Apricots, canned with syrup	30	0.1	0	3.4		A
Apricots, dried	52	1.4	0	12.3		A
Apricots, fresh	12	0.2	Tr	3.9		A
Avocado pear	24	0.4	3.1	2.5		C
Banana	22	0.3	0	5.5		
Blackberries	8	0.4	Tr	1.8		C
Blackcurrants	8	0.3	0	1.9		C
Blueberries, canned, sweet	25	Tr	Tr	6.9		C
Cherries	14	0.2	0	3.4		
Cherries, canned with syrup	36	0.2	0	3.4		A
Cranberry sauce, canned, sweet	50	Tr	Tr	12.9		
Dates, dried	70	0.6	0	18.1		
Dates, fresh	70	0.6	Tr	18.1		
Figs, canned in syrup	22	0.4	Tr	4.2		
Figs, dried	60	1.0	0	15.0		

FOOD	Calories	Protein g	Fat g	Carbohy-drate g	Reliable Mineral Source	Reliable Vitamin Source
Figs, fresh	12	0.4	Tr	2.7		
Gooseberries	8	0.3	0	1.8		C
Grapefruit	6	0.2	0	1.5		C
Grapes	15	0.4	0.3	4.2		
Guava	17	0.3	Tr	4.0		
Lemon	2	0.1	0	0.5		C
Mandarin	8	0.1	0	1.8		C
Mandarin, canned with syrup	18	0.1	0	4.7		C
Mango	36	0.5	Tr	4.8		
Melon	6	0.2	0	1.5		A
Olives	30	0.3	3.1	Tr		
Orange	10	0.2	0	2.4		C
Orange juice, canned, unconcentrated	13	0.2	0	3.3		C
Passion fruit	10	0.8	Tr	1.8		
Peaches, canned inc. syrup	25	0.1	0	6.5		A
Peaches, fresh	11	0.2	0	3.3		A
Pears, fresh	12	0.1	0	3.0		
Pineapple, canned inc. syrup	22	0.1	0	5.7		
Pineapple, fresh	13	0.1	0	2.3		C
Plums	9	0.2	0	2.2		
Prunes, canned	33	0.2	0	6.8		
Prunes, dried	46	0.7	0	11.4		A
Raisins	80	0.4	0	21.0		
Raspberries	7	0.3	0	1.6		C
Rhubarb	2	0.2	0	0.3		
Rhubarb, canned with syrup	24	0.2	0	3.3		
Strawberries	8	0.2	0	1.8		C
Strawberries, canned with syrup	18	0.2	0	3.6		
Sultanas	71	0.5	0	18.3		

Nuts

Almonds	170	5.8	15.2	1.2	Calcium, Phosphorus	B, E

FOOD	Calories	Protein g	Fat g	Carbohydrate g	Reliable Mineral Source	Reliable Vitamin Source
Almonds, roast	176	5.0	13.9	5.5		B, E
Almonds, roasted and salted	178	5.0	13.9	5.5		
Brazil	183	3.9	17.3	1.2	Calcium, Phosphorus	B, E
Cashews	159	5.0	12.5	8.3		
Cashews, salted	157	5.0	12.5	8.3		
Chestnuts	49	0.7	0.8	10.4		B
Cob	113	2.6	10.2	1.9		B
Coconut	104	1.1	10.2	1.9		B
Coconut, dried	178	1.9	17.6	1.8		B
Hazelnuts	181	3.1	10.2	1.2		B
Peanuts	171	8.0	13.9	2.4	Calcium	B, E
Peanuts, salted	175	6.9	11.6	3.4		
Pecans, dry, roasted	195	2.6	19.2	4.1		
Pistachios	155	5	13.5	0		A, B
Walnuts	156	3.6	14.6	1.4	Calcium	B

Dairy produce

FOOD	Calories	Protein g	Fat g	Carbohydrate g	Reliable Mineral Source	Reliable Vitamin Source
Buttermilk	10	0.9	Tr	1.4	Calcium, Phosphorus	
Cream, double [thick]	127	0.5	13.6	0.7	Calcium, Phosphorus	A, B
Cream, single [thin]	54	0.8	5.1	1.2	Calcium, Phosphorus	A, B
Custard	92	3.0	3.5	12.9	Calcium	B
Goat's milk	20	0.9	1.2	1.3	Calcium, Phosphorus	A, B
Milk	19	0.9	1.1	1.4	Calcium, Phosphorus	A, B
Milk, condensed, sweetened	91	2.3	2.6	15.6	Calcium, Phosphorus	A, B
Milk, dried, skimmed	100	10.2	0.3	5.2	Calcium, Phosphorus	B
Milk, evaporated	46	2.4	2.6	3.6	Calcium, Phosphorus	A, B
Yoghurt, low fat, fruit	28	1.4	0.3	5.2	Calcium, Phosphorus	B
Yoghurt, low fat, natural	15	1.4	0.3	1.8	Calcium, Phosphorus	B

FOOD	Calories	Protein g	Fat g	Carbohy-drate g	Reliable Mineral Source	Reliable Vitamin Source
Cheese						
Camembert	88	6.5	6.6	Tr		A, B, E
Cheddar	117	7.2	9.8	0	Calcium, Phosphorus	A, B, E
Cheshire	110	7.3	8.7	Tr	Calcium, Phosphorus	A, B, E
Cottage	32	4.3	1.1	1.3	Phosphorus	B, E
Cream	232	0.9	24.5	Tr	Calcium, Phosphorus	A, B, E
Danish Blue	103	6.5	8.3	Tr	Calcium, Phosphorus	A, B, E
Edam	88	6.9	6.5	Tr	Calcium, Phosphorus	A, B, E
Gorgonzola	112	7.2	8.8	Tr	Calcium, Phosphorus	A, B, E
Gouda	96	6.3	7.6	Tr	Calcium, Phosphorus	A, B, E
Gruyere	132	10.7	9.5	Tr	Calcium, Phosphorus	A, B, E
Parmesan	118	7.1	6.3	0.7	Calcium, Phosphorus	A, B, E
Processed	106	6.5	8.5	Tr	Calcium, Phosphorus	A, B, E
Spread	82	5.1	6.5	Tr	Calcium, Phosphorus	A, B, E
Stilton	135	7.3	11.4	Tr	Calcium, Phosphorus	A, B, E
Fat & oil						
Butter	207	0.1	23.0	0		A, D, E
Coconut oil	265	0	30.0	0		
Dripping, lard, cooking fat	254	0	28.2	0		
French dressing	170	0.2	15.0	7.5		
Low-fat spread	103	0	11.5	0		A, D
Margarine	208	0.1	23.1	0		A, D
Mayonnaise	280	0.4	30.0	0.8	Iron	A, B, D, E
Olive oil	270	0	30.0	0		
Suet	254	0.46	28.0	0		A
Sunflower oil	270	0	30.0	0		E

FOOD	Calories	Protein g	Fat g	Carbohy-drate g	Reliable Mineral Source	Reliable Vitamin Source
Eggs						
Fresh, boiled	42	3.4	3.1	0	Iron	A, B, D, E
Fried	68	4.0	5.5	Tr	Iron	A, B, D, E
Poached	45	3.5	3.3	Tr	Iron	A, B, D, E
Egg white	11	2.6	Tr	Tr		
Egg yolk	99	4.6	8.7	Tr	Iron	A, B, D, E
Duck egg	41	2.8	3.2	Tr	Iron	A, B, D, E
Cereals						
Barley, cooked	34	0.7	0.2	7.8		
Bran cereal	88	3.6	1.3	16.5	Iron	B
Breadcrumbs	101	3.3	0.5	22.0	Calcium, Iron	B
Bread, currant, raisin	71	1.8	1.0	14.7	Calcium	B
Bread, malt	71	1.8	1.0	14.7	Calcium	B
Bread, starch-reduced	66	3.0	0.4	13.5	Calcium, Iron	B
Bread, white	72	2.3	0.5	15.4	Calcium, Iron	B
Bread, white, fried	162	2.1	10.6	14.6	Calcium, Iron	B
Bread, white, toast	85	2.7	0.5	18.4	Calcium, Iron	B
Bread, wholemeal	68	2.7	0.9	13.2	Iron	B, E
Cornflakes	100	2.1	0.1	24.2		B
Cornflour [Cornstarch]	100	0.1	0.2	26.2	Iron	
Egg noodles, boiled	18	0.6	Tr	4		
Flour, rye	85	2	0.5	20		B
Flour, white	99	2.8	0.3	22.7	Calcium, Iron	B
Flour, wholemeal	96	3.0	0.3	22.8	Iron, Calcium	B
Macaroni, boiled	32	1.0	0.2	7.2	Calcium, Iron	B
Matzomeal	125	2.8	Tr	30.6	Calcium, Iron	B
Muesli	120	1.5	5.4	0.6	Calcium	B
Porridge (oatmeal)	13	0.4	0.3	2.3	Calcium, Iron	B
Porridge boiled with water	13	0.4	0.3	2.3		
Rice, boiled	35	0.6	0.1	8.4		
Rice, brown, cooked	35	1.8	0.3	24.6		B
Rice, puffed	102	1.6	0.3	24.2	Iron	B

FOOD	Calories	Protein g	Fat g	Carbohy-drate g	Reliable Mineral Source	Reliable Vitamin Source
Soya flour	123	11.5	6.7	3.8		
Spaghetti, boiled	32	2.8	0.3	23.8	Calcium, Iron	B
Wheat, puffed	100	3.1	0.5	21.9	Iron	B
Wheat, shredded	103	2.8	0.8	22.4	Iron	B

Biscuits and Cakes

FOOD	Calories	Protein g	Fat g	Carbohy-drate g	Reliable Mineral Source	Reliable Vitamin Source
Cheese straws	172	4.7	13.5	7.3		
Chocolate biscuits [cookies]	141	2.0	7.1	18.5		
Cream crackers, plain	134	2.3	4.6	22.1		
Crispbread	90	2.8	0.6	19.6		
Digestive [Graham crackers]	137	2.7	5.8	18.7		
Matzos	125	2.8	Tr	30.6	Calcium, Iron	B
Muffins	70	2.0	2.2	9.6		
Plain, dry biscuits	123	2.1	3.8	21.4		
Rye wafers	84	3.5	0.3	20.1		
Shortbread	150	1.8	5.4	16.2		
Sweet	50	1.2	4.1	18.2		
Wafer biscuits	127	2.7	4.6	19.4		
Water biscuits	126	3.0	3.5	20.7		

Puddings, pastries and cakes

FOOD	Calories	Protein g	Fat g	Carbohy-drate g	Reliable Mineral Source	Reliable Vitamin Source
Apple pie	80	0.9	4.1	11.5		
Blancmange	35	1.0	0.9	5.2	Calcium	A, B (if made with milk)
Bread and butter pudding	44	1.6	2.0	5.2	Calcium	B
Buns, currant	93	2.2	2.4	16.6		B
Chocolate cake	130	1.9	6.3	24	Iron	
Christmas [Plum] Pudding	92	1.4	4.1	12.9		
Doughnut	120	2.0	6.5	13		
Fruit cake	105	2.0	6.2	23		
Fruit crumble	80	0.9	4.1	11.5		
Ice cream	53	1.2	3.2	5.6	Calcium	B
Jam tarts	111	0.9	3.9	19.2		

FOOD	Calories	Protein g	Fat g	Carbohydrate g	Reliable Mineral Source	Reliable Vitamin Source
Jelly, fruit	34	1.0	0	5.9		
Jelly, plain	23	0.6	0	5.4		
Meringue	110	0.9	0	27		
Mince pie	90	0.6	3.1	10.1		
Pastry	176	2	13.2	16		
Rice pudding	41	1.0	2.2	4.5	Calcium	B
Scones	105	2.2	3.7	16.3		
Sponge cake	100	3	2	17		
Trifle	46	0.9	1.6	7.5	Calcium	B
Waffles	71	2.1	2.5	9.8		
Yorkshire pudding	65	2	2.8	8	Phosphorus	

Sugars, sweets and candies

FOOD	Calories	Protein g	Fat g	Carbohydrate g	Reliable Mineral Source	Reliable Vitamin Source
Boiled sweets	43	0.1	Tr	11.4		
Butterscotch	120	0	2.8	17		
Cherries, glace	60	0.2	0	15.8		
Chocolate, milk	167	2.5	10.7	15.5	Calcium	
Chocolate, plain	155	1.6	10.0	14.9	Iron	
Fruit gums	49	0.3	0	12.7		
Fudge	130	0.5	3.0	21.2		
Honeycomb	80	0.2	1.3	21.2		
Honey	82	0.1	Tr	21.7		
Liquid glucose	90	Tr	0	24.1		
Liquorice	90	1.1	0.6	21.0		
Peanut brittle	129	2.5	4.0	18.9	Calcium	B
Peppermints	111	0.1	0.2	29.0		
Popcorn	103	3.5	1.5	20.3		
Sugar, brown	112	0.1	0	29.6		
Sugar, white	112	Tr	0	29.7		
Syrup, golden	84	0.1	0	22.4		
Toffee, homemade	113	0.1	1.8	25.6		
Toffees, mixed	123	0.6	4.9	20.2		
Treacle, black [molasses]	73	0.3	0	19.1	Potassium	

FOOD	Calories	Protein g	Fat g	Carbohy-drate g	Reliable Mineral Source	Reliable Vitamin Source
Condiments and preserves						
Chutney, apple	57	0.2	Tr	14.8		
Chutney, tomato	43	0.3	Tr	11.0		
Curry powder	67	2.7	3.1	7.4		
Ginger, ground	74	2.1	0.9	17.0		
Jam, fruit with edible seeds	74	0.2	0	19.6		
Lemon curd	86	0.9	3.9	12.0		
Marmalade	74	Tr	0	19.8		C
Mincemeat	37	0.2	0.9	7.2		
Mustard	132	8.2	8.1	5.9		
Peanut butter	175	6.9	12.2	4.9		
Pepper	88	2.5	1.8	19.3		
Pickles, mustard	70	0.3	0.2	1.0		
Pickles, sweet	36.1	Tr	Tr	9.0		
Salt	0	0	0	0		
Sauce, brown	33	0.8	2.2	2.5		
Sauce, tomato (catsup)	21	0.7	1.1	2.1		
Vinegar	1.0	0.1	0	0.2		
Yeast extract	2	0.4	Tr	0	Calcium, Iron Potassium	B
Liquids **Hot drinks** (per 225ml [8oz] cupful)						
Instant coffee, black	2	0	0	1		
Instant coffee with 30ml [2tbs] milk	20	0.9	1.1	2.4		
Instant coffee with milk and 10ml [2tsp] sugar	97	0.9	1.1	22.4		
Cocoa made with milk	160	10.3	9.9	11	Iron	A, B
Cocoa made with milk and 10ml [2tsp] sugar	235	10.3	9.9	31	Iron	A, B
Chocolate made with milk	175	8.2	9.9	21	Calcium	B
Chocolate made with milk and 10ml [2tsp] sugar	250	8.2	9.9	41	Calcium	B
Malted drinks made with milk	185	8.2	9.9	22		
Malted drinks made with milk and 10ml [2tsp] sugar	260	8.2	9.9	42		

LIQUIDS	Calories	Protein g	Fat g	Carbohydrate g	Reliable Mineral Source	Reliable Vitamin Source
Tea, black	0	0	0	0		
Tea, with 30ml [2tbs] milk	20	0.9	1.1	1.4		
Tea, milk and 10ml [2tsp] sugar	95	0.9	1.1	1.4		

Fruit juice (per 150ml [5oz] glass)

Grapefruit	55	0.7	0	14		C
Lemon, unsweetened	10	Tr	Tr	3		C
Orange	60	1.0	0	16		C
Pineapple	70	0.5	0	18		
Tomato	25	1.0	0.2	5		C

Soft drinks (per 320ml [11½oz] can, unless otherwise stated)

Bitter lemon	110	Tr	Tr	28		
Blackcurrant, concentrated, 15ml [1tbs]	35	0.05	0	10		C
Cola	150	0	0	39		
Dry ginger	50	0	0	12		
Fizzy lemonade, 570ml [20oz]	120	Tr	0	32		
Tonic water	94	0	0	24		

Alcohol

Brown ale, 570ml [20oz]	160	1.4	Tr	16.8		
Draught bitter, 570ml [20oz]	180	1.4	Tr	12.8		
Lager, 570ml [20oz]	150	0	0	16.9		
Pale ale, 570ml [20oz]	180	0	0	11.2		
Stout, 570ml [20oz]	200	16.2	Tr	52		
Brandy, 24ml [gill]	75	0	0	Tr		
Gin, 24ml [gill]	53	0	0	Tr		
Port, 50ml [gill]	76	0	0	3.24		
Rum, 24ml [gill]	53	0	0	Tr		
Vodka, 24ml [gill]	53	0	0	Tr		
Whisky, 24ml [gill]	53	0	0	Tr		
Wine, red, 110ml [4oz]	76	0	0	0.3		
Wine, white, dry, 110ml [4oz]	84	0	0	1.6		
Wine, white, sweet, 110ml [4oz]	96	0	0	6.7		

EXERCISE TO ELEGANCE
MADE TO MEASURE

If you are seriously interested in keeping your body in trim, you must accept that some kind of regular exercise is necessary to tone and tighten flabby muscles.

This exercise routine can be done at home, in less than half an hour per day and it requires no special equipment or expenditure, save that of your own energy! But do not make the mistake of thinking that these exercises alone will make you lose weight, because they will not. You must practise them in conjunction with a sensible diet if you want to shed pounds. However, provided you follow the instructions carefully, the exercises will help tone specific areas of your body that need attention, making you look better and feel fitter.

An exercise routine should become a regular habit. First thing in the morning is a good time to choose. Alternatively, you could break your exercise routine into two sessions and slot them into convenient times of the day. The important thing is to remember to make the routines regular. They need not be followed every single day, but do try to have at least three or four sessions a week.

Never exercise immediately after meals, otherwise you could end up with cramps, discomfort and indigestion. Choose minimal, light clothes and keep the room cool because you will work up a certain amount of body heat while doing your exercises. A bath after an exercise session will leave you feeling completely relaxed and healthily refreshed.

It is important to read the instructions for each exercise very carefully before trying it out—it is surprisingly easy to get an exercise wrong and make useless gestures that are not using the muscles at all. You may need to do quite a lot of practise at first to get it right, so don't try to work too hard when you begin: concentrate rather on getting each exercise performed smoothly and carefully.

The emphasis should be on strength, not strain. If at first you can't manage the whole set of movements involved in any particular exercise, you should aim steadily towards it, following the correct procedure. Exercises that may seem very difficult at first soon begin to feel easier as your body adjusts to the extra work, and the muscles become stronger and more supple.

To do any good, an exercise routine must be *progressive*. You constantly need to pace yourself to begin with, because as an exercise becomes easier, so

you must do more repetitions in order to gain the maximum effect. But this isn't to say that you will be doing exercises into infinity! You never need spend more than half an hour at any exercise session, and you can build into it those exercises that you feel are needed for your body.

For this reason, the exercises are divided into six sessions, each one devoted to a different area of the body, so you can choose the ones you feel your body needs. The first section is a general, warming up routine, which everyone should follow. The last section is a gentle, 'winding down' relaxation routine which is quite optional, but makes a good conclusion to the workout. Otherwise, the choice is yours, and a suggestion would be to do two exercises from each section to begin with, and then concentrate on the particular areas of your body that you would most like to see trimmed down.

Correct breathing is important. Although fairly strenuous, none of the exercises is so energetic that it has a major influence on your pulse rate, but nevertheless you may find yourself out of breath quite quickly, particularly if you are very unfit to start off with.

Spend some time before starting to exercise in deep, proper breathing from the diaphragm, and inhale slowly through the nose, exhaling sharply through the mouth. You will need to stand with your hands on your ribs to do this, to check that the diaphragm and lower part of the lungs are being properly filled with air, and that you're not breathing only with the top part of your lungs. If, during your exercise workout, you find yourself getting very out of breath, stop for a minute and do this simple breathing exercise. You should never wind up a session absolutely exhausted.

None of the exercises should harm you, however little you are used to exercise, provided you go about them in the right way. Never start a session completely 'cold', as this is the way muscles and tendons can get pulled and strained. Always begin with a five minute warm up session and if you are feeling particularly cold and stiff, add a one minute running on the spot exercise too. If you suffer from rheumatism, arthritis, or have suffered any joint or spinal injury, it does make sense to check with your doctor before starting an exercise programme, and the same goes for anyone receiving any kind of medical treatment.

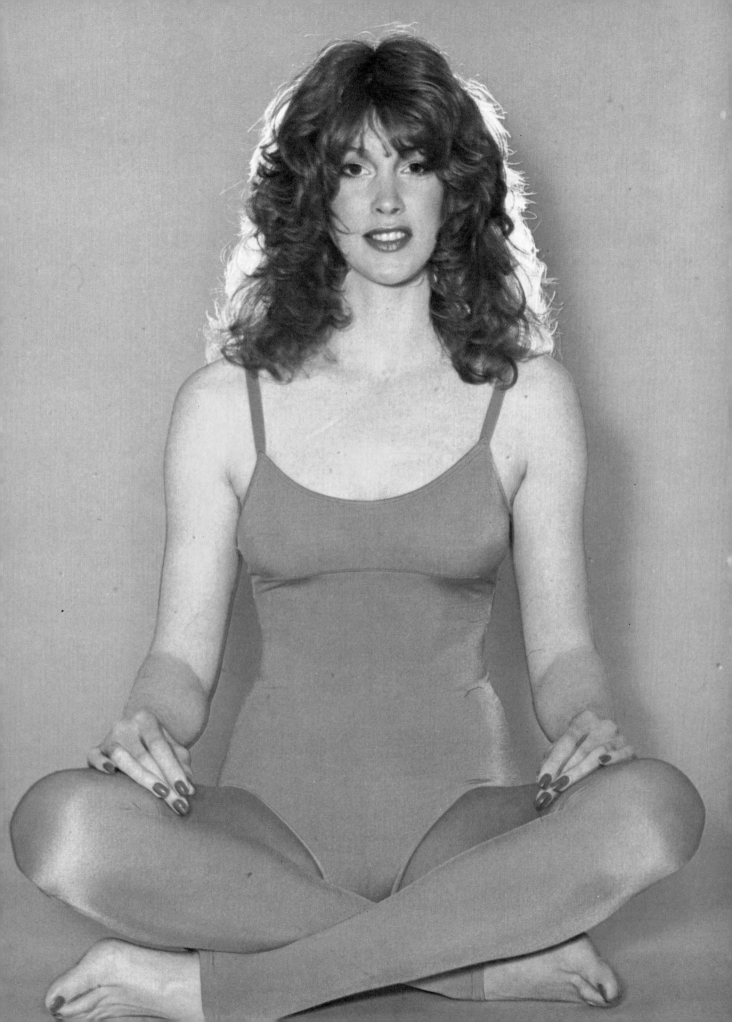

WARMING UP

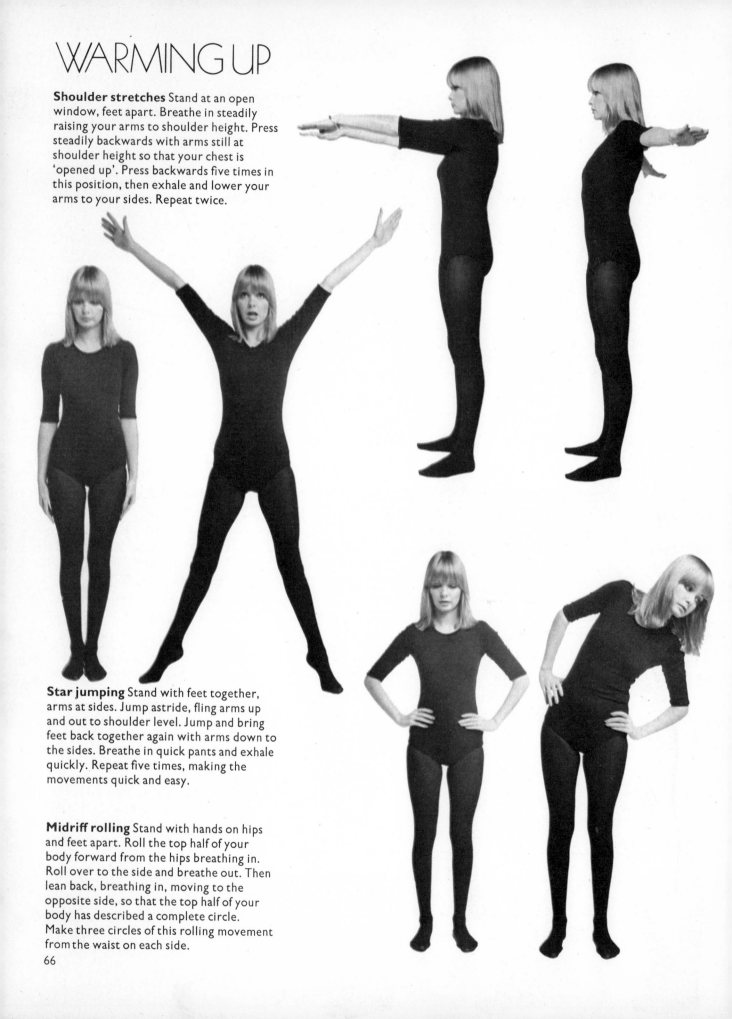

Shoulder stretches Stand at an open window, feet apart. Breathe in steadily raising your arms to shoulder height. Press steadily backwards with arms still at shoulder height so that your chest is 'opened up'. Press backwards five times in this position, then exhale and lower your arms to your sides. Repeat twice.

Star jumping Stand with feet together, arms at sides. Jump astride, fling arms up and out to shoulder level. Jump and bring feet back together again with arms down to the sides. Breathe in quick pants and exhale quickly. Repeat five times, making the movements quick and easy.

Midriff rolling Stand with hands on hips and feet apart. Roll the top half of your body forward from the hips breathing in. Roll over to the side and breathe out. Then lean back, breathing in, moving to the opposite side, so that the top half of your body has described a complete circle. Make three circles of this rolling movement from the waist on each side.

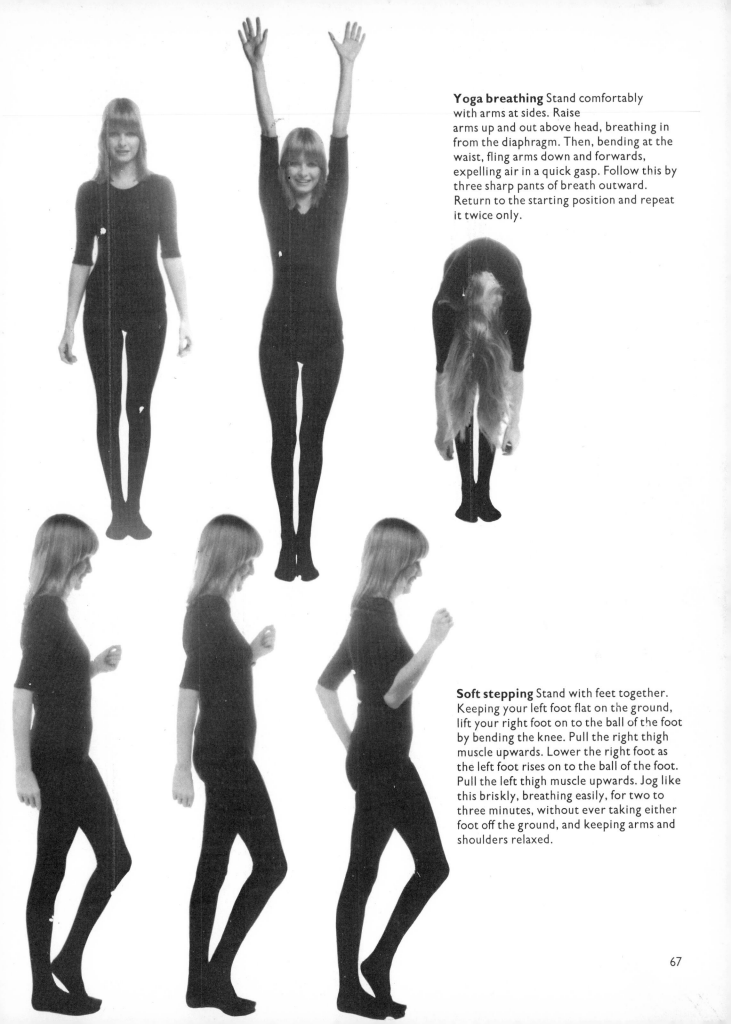

Yoga breathing Stand comfortably
with arms at sides. Raise
arms up and out above head, breathing in
from the diaphragm. Then, bending at the
waist, fling arms down and forwards,
expelling air in a quick gasp. Follow this by
three sharp pants of breath outward.
Return to the starting position and repeat
it twice only.

Soft stepping Stand with feet together.
Keeping your left foot flat on the ground,
lift your right foot on to the ball of the foot
by bending the knee. Pull the right thigh
muscle upwards. Lower the right foot as
the left foot rises on to the ball of the foot.
Pull the left thigh muscle upwards. Jog like
this briskly, breathing easily, for two to
three minutes, without ever taking either
foot off the ground, and keeping arms and
shoulders relaxed.

ARMS AND SHOULDERS

Kneel-ups Squat on hands and knees, with arms straight and thighs vertical. Breathe in and bend your arms to bring your chin down to touch the floor, breathe out and press up again until your arms are straight. Do this twice only, progressing in twos as you become more proficient.

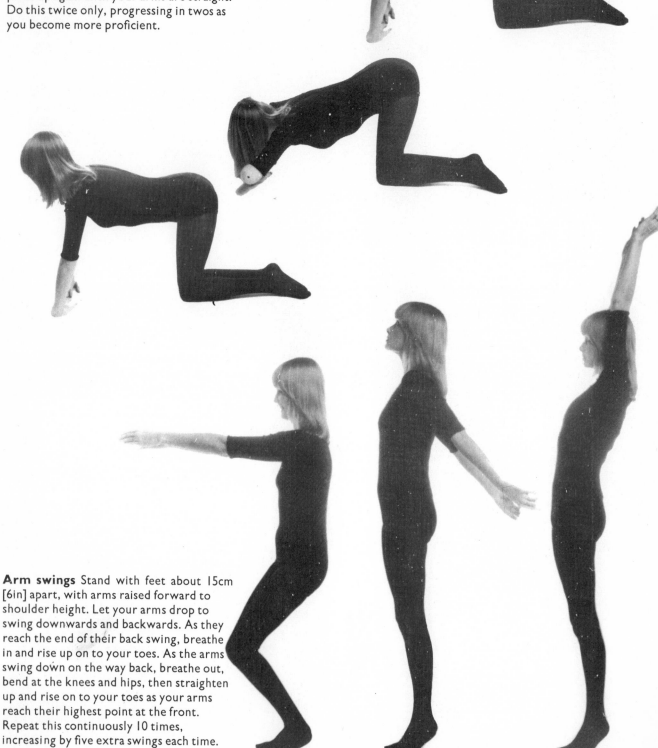

Arm swings Stand with feet about 15cm [6in] apart, with arms raised forward to shoulder height. Let your arms drop to swing downwards and backwards. As they reach the end of their back swing, breathe in and rise up on to your toes. As the arms swing down on the way back, breathe out, bend at the knees and hips, then straighten up and rise on to your toes as your arms reach their highest point at the front. Repeat this continuously 10 times, increasing by five extra swings each time.

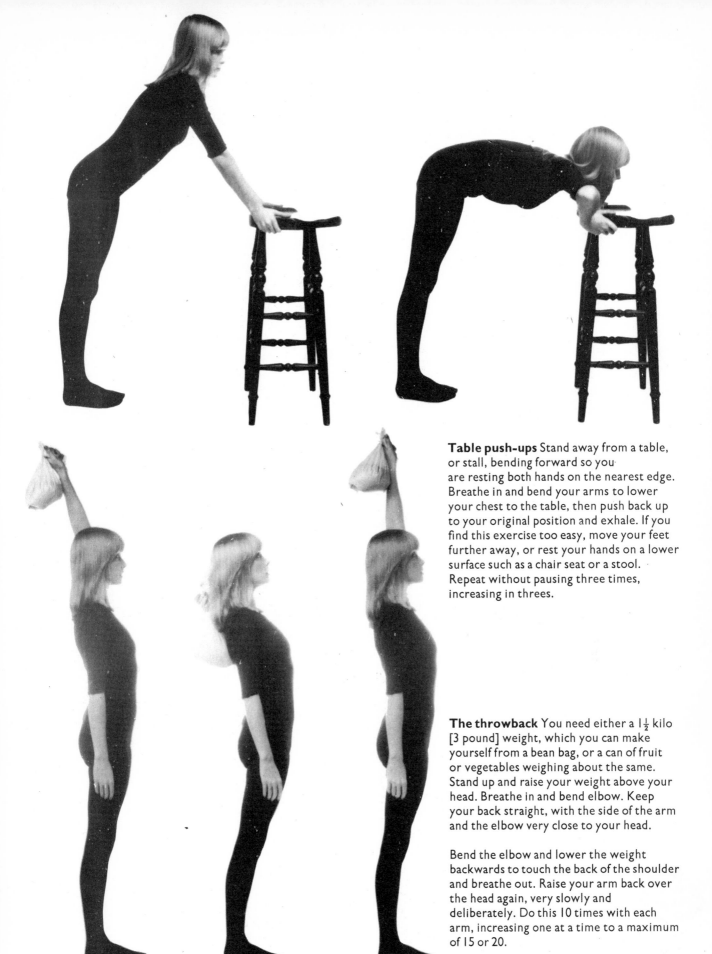

Table push-ups Stand away from a table, or stall, bending forward so you are resting both hands on the nearest edge. Breathe in and bend your arms to lower your chest to the table, then push back up to your original position and exhale. If you find this exercise too easy, move your feet further away, or rest your hands on a lower surface such as a chair seat or a stool. Repeat without pausing three times, increasing in threes.

The throwback You need either a $1\frac{1}{2}$ kilo [3 pound] weight, which you can make yourself from a bean bag, or a can of fruit or vegetables weighing about the same. Stand up and raise your weight above your head. Breathe in and bend elbow. Keep your back straight, with the side of the arm and the elbow very close to your head.

Bend the elbow and lower the weight backwards to touch the back of the shoulder and breathe out. Raise your arm back over the head again, very slowly and deliberately. Do this 10 times with each arm, increasing one at a time to a maximum of 15 or 20.

BUST AND BACK

Arm crossing Stand with arms held out at shoulder level, fingers stretched and palms facing forward. Inhale and swing your arms across the chest, bouncing them twice very firmly, trying to squeeze your chest inwards. Keep elbows straight, and swing your arms out to the sides again. Exhale, then drop your arms to your sides firmly, with palms facing back. Bounce the arms twice backwards, keeping fingers stretched and fingers and arms rigid. Relax, then go into the exercise again, repeating it ten times. Build up to 15, then 20.

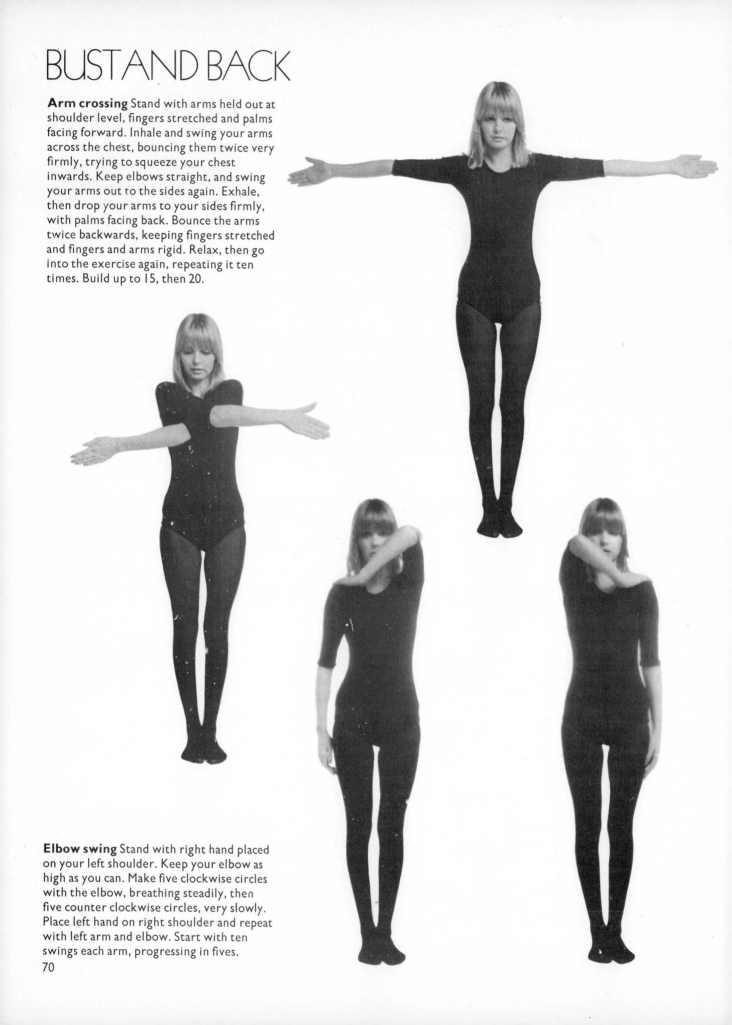

Elbow swing Stand with right hand placed on your left shoulder. Keep your elbow as high as you can. Make five clockwise circles with the elbow, breathing steadily, then five counter clockwise circles, very slowly. Place left hand on right shoulder and repeat with left arm and elbow. Start with ten swings each arm, progressing in fives.

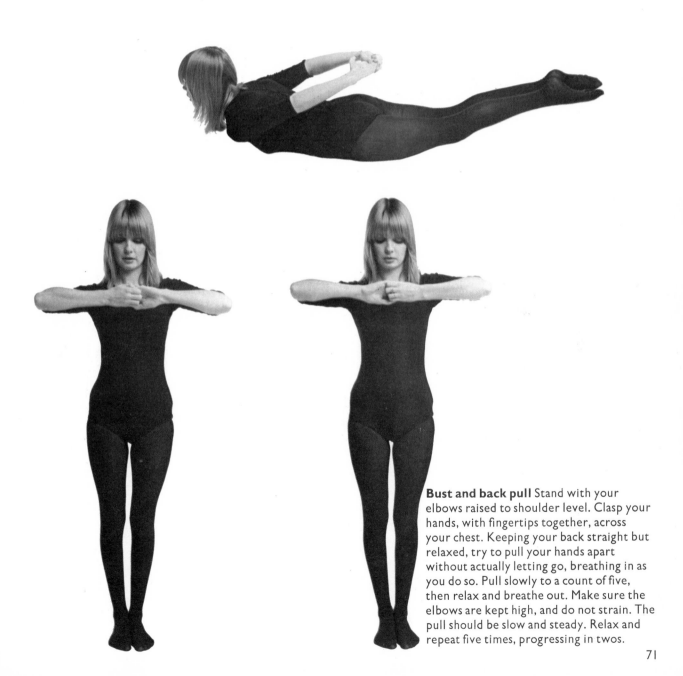

Back raises Lie flat on your face with your hands clasped behind your back. Raise your head and legs away from the floor. Breathe in as you do so. Hold your head and legs up and still, briefly, and then lower them gently. Continue to do this steadily, repeating it 10 times and progressing in fives.

Bust and back pull Stand with your elbows raised to shoulder level. Clasp your hands, with fingertips together, across your chest. Keeping your back straight but relaxed, try to pull your hands apart without actually letting go, breathing in as you do so. Pull slowly to a count of five, then relax and breathe out. Make sure the elbows are kept high, and do not strain. The pull should be slow and steady. Relax and repeat five times, progressing in twos.

WAIST AND MIDRIFF

Side arches Sit on your left side, with legs straight along the floor and one foot slightly in front of the other. Support yourself on your left arm. Keep your right arm at your side. Breathe in and raise your hips from the floor and arch them sideways high into the air, supporting your weight on your left arm and both feet. Lower and exhale. Repeat 10 times to the left and 10 times to the right for one complete set.

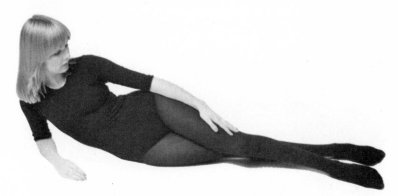

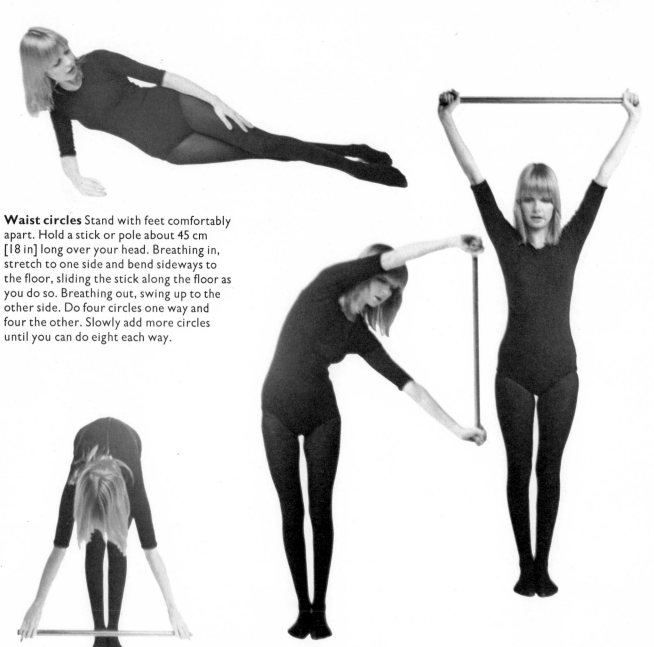

Waist circles Stand with feet comfortably apart. Hold a stick or pole about 45 cm [18 in] long over your head. Breathing in, stretch to one side and bend sideways to the floor, sliding the stick along the floor as you do so. Breathing out, swing up to the other side. Do four circles one way and four the other. Slowly add more circles until you can do eight each way.

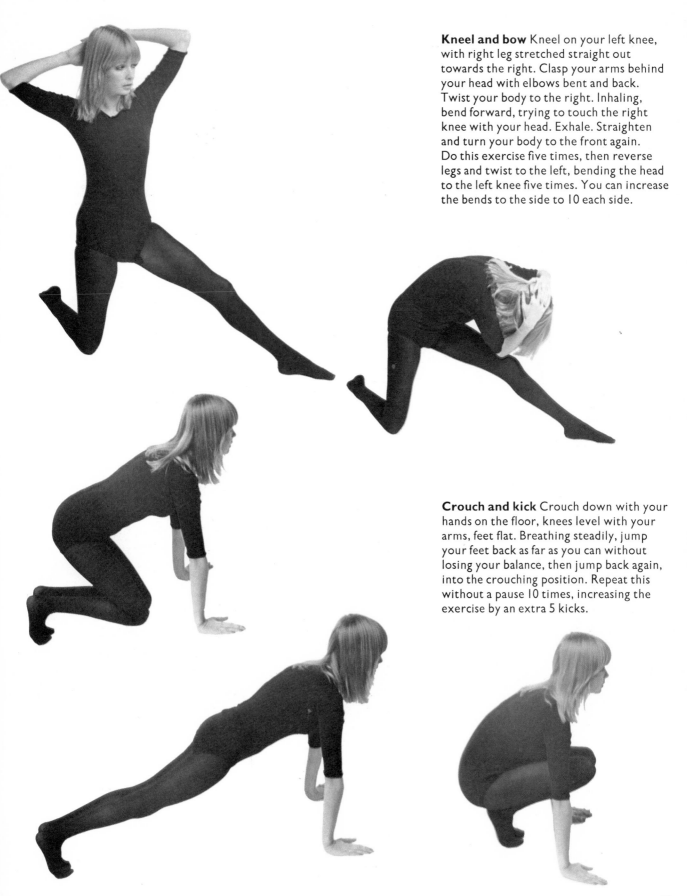

Kneel and bow Kneel on your left knee, with right leg stretched straight out towards the right. Clasp your arms behind your head with elbows bent and back. Twist your body to the right. Inhaling, bend forward, trying to touch the right knee with your head. Exhale. Straighten and turn your body to the front again. Do this exercise five times, then reverse legs and twist to the left, bending the head to the left knee five times. You can increase the bends to the side to 10 each side.

Crouch and kick Crouch down with your hands on the floor, knees level with your arms, feet flat. Breathing steadily, jump your feet back as far as you can without losing your balance, then jump back again, into the crouching position. Repeat this without a pause 10 times, increasing the exercise by an extra 5 kicks.

STOMACH

Leg roll! Lie flat on your back on the floor. Spread your arms out sideways, breathe in and raise both legs into the air until your thighs are straight, at right angles to your body. You may need to bend the knees slightly at first. Breathe out and roll the legs down sideways to touch the floor at the left side, then raise them up again without pausing and carry them over and down at the other side. Repeat this movement five times, increasing by five for each set.

Leg tucks Lie flat on your back on the floor with arms held close to your sides. Take a deep breath, then raise one knee up to your chin. Pull it in to your chest tightly with your arms. Breathe out. Then, slowly and in time with your breathing, change over legs and continue without stopping until you have done this five times with each leg. Increase by three movements as you progress.

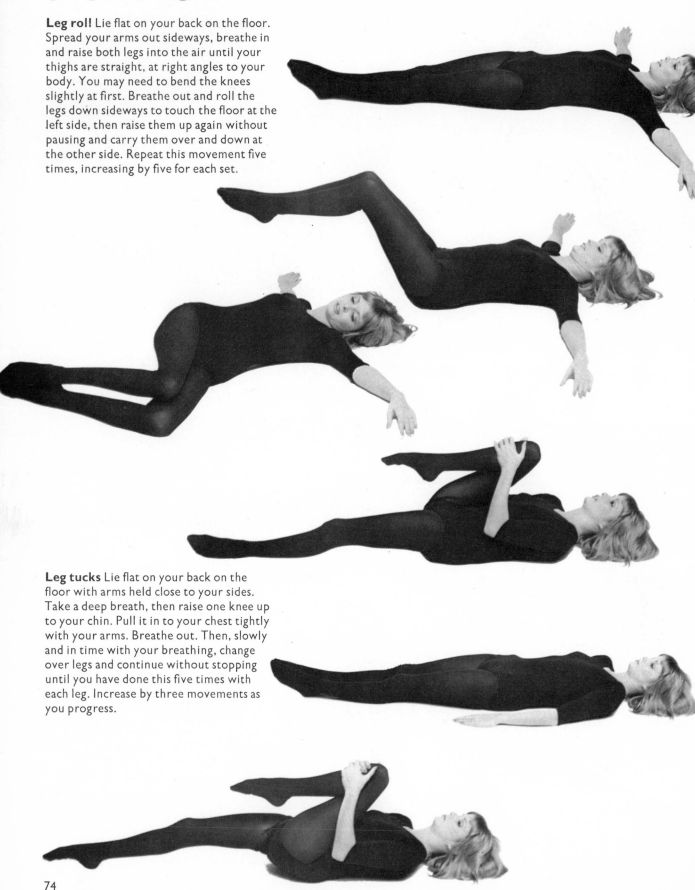

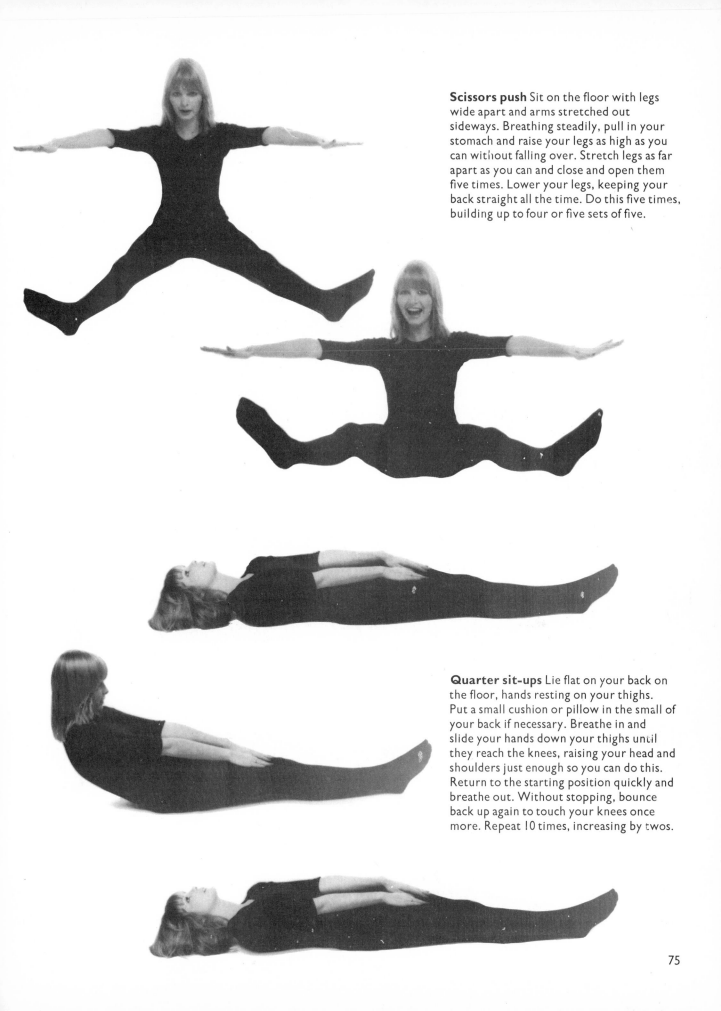

Scissors push Sit on the floor with legs wide apart and arms stretched out sideways. Breathing steadily, pull in your stomach and raise your legs as high as you can without falling over. Stretch legs as far apart as you can and close and open them five times. Lower your legs, keeping your back straight all the time. Do this five times, building up to four or five sets of five.

Quarter sit-ups Lie flat on your back on the floor, hands resting on your thighs. Put a small cushion or pillow in the small of your back if necessary. Breathe in and slide your hands down your thighs until they reach the knees, raising your head and shoulders just enough so you can do this. Return to the starting position quickly and breathe out. Without stopping, bounce back up again to touch your knees once more. Repeat 10 times, increasing by twos.

BOTTOM
AND HIPS

Foot fling Get down on all fours. Breathe in and raise your right leg and kick up backwards as high as possible, quite briskly 10 times. Breathing out, return to the all fours position and raise the left leg and kick up backwards 10 times. Increase by one to a maximum of 20.

Bottom bounce Sit with your legs out in front, straight and together, with hands behind for support. Bend the right knee and place your right foot by your left calf. Turn your left foot towards the floor. Using the right foot as a lever lift seat and breathe in, taking your weight on your hands and bounce on the outside on the left buttock twice breathing out. Return to the legs straight out position. Bend the left knee and place the left foot by the right calf. Turn the right foot towards the floor. Return the right foot to the toes-up position and bounce twice on the outside of the right buttock. Do this exercise fast and briskly 10 times, working up gradually to 20 times.

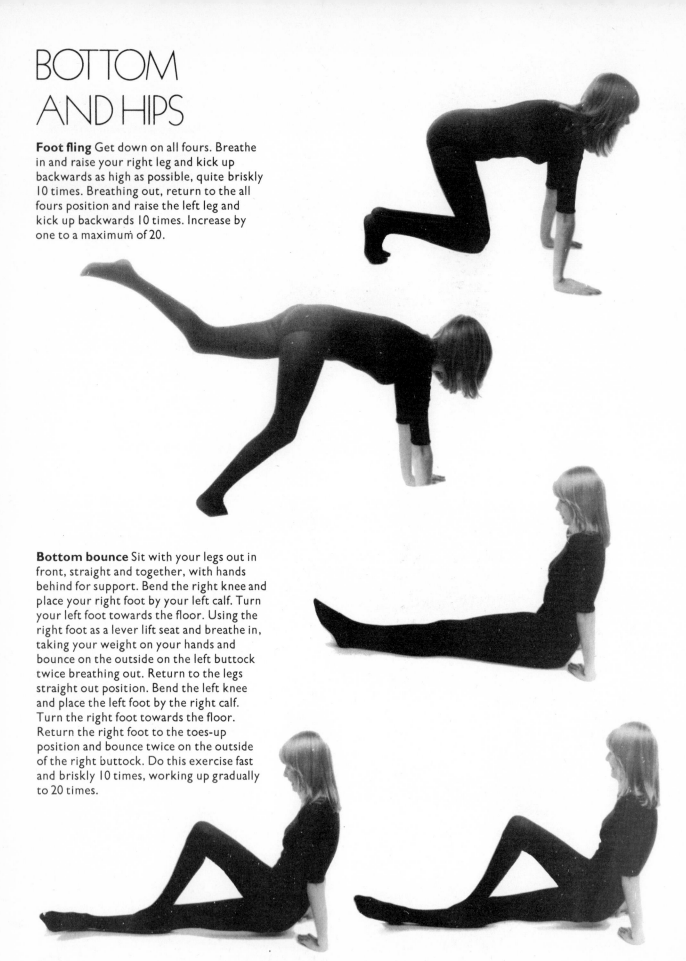

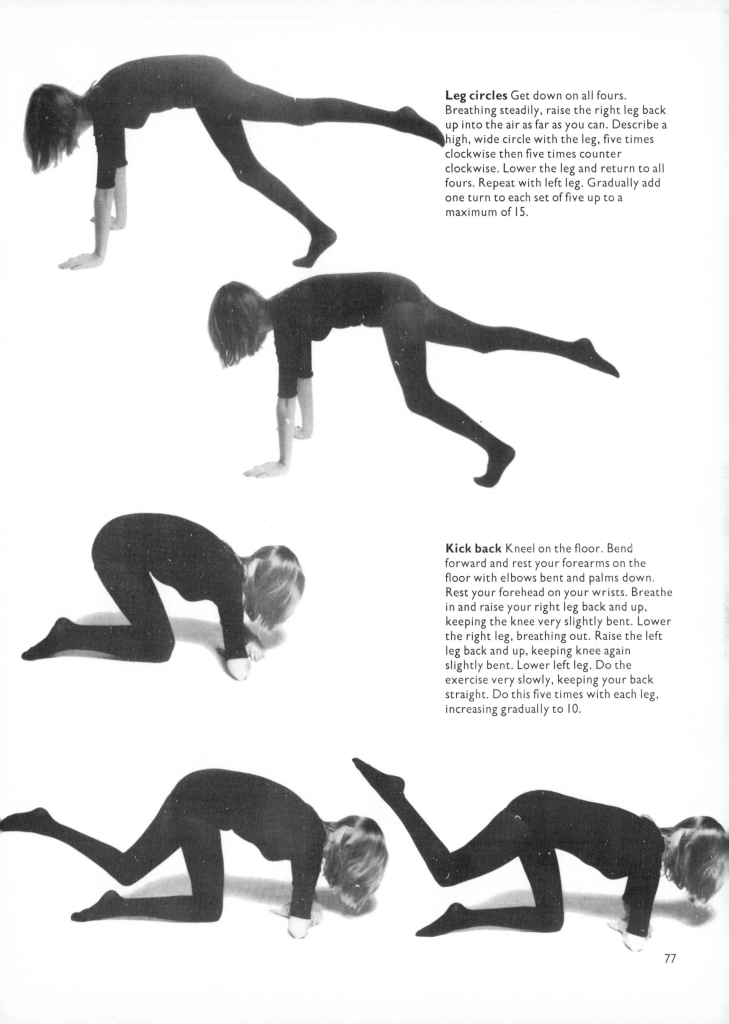

Leg circles Get down on all fours. Breathing steadily, raise the right leg back up into the air as far as you can. Describe a high, wide circle with the leg, five times clockwise then five times counter clockwise. Lower the leg and return to all fours. Repeat with left leg. Gradually add one turn to each set of five up to a maximum of 15.

Kick back Kneel on the floor. Bend forward and rest your forearms on the floor with elbows bent and palms down. Rest your forehead on your wrists. Breathe in and raise your right leg back and up, keeping the knee very slightly bent. Lower the right leg, breathing out. Raise the left leg back and up, keeping knee again slightly bent. Lower left leg. Do the exercise very slowly, keeping your back straight. Do this five times with each leg, increasing gradually to 10.

LEGS AND ANKLES

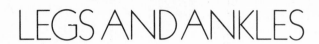

High knee raising Stand and keep your eyes fixed on any convenient mark that is about 10 cm [4 in] above eye level. Breathing steadily run on the spot, raising your knees to waist height. Bounce on each step so that your eyes become level with the mark you've chosen.

Thigh slapping Sit on the floor with your arms resting behind your body for support. Breathe in and bend the right knee so that the right foot slides up to the left knee. Keeping the right knee bent, push the right leg out sideways, breathing out, so that the outside of the right thigh slaps the floor. Bring the right leg back to the upright position. Slap the right leg straight down on the floor, then return to starting position. Repeat these movements with the left leg and do the movements 10 times each leg, working up in fives to a maximum of 30.

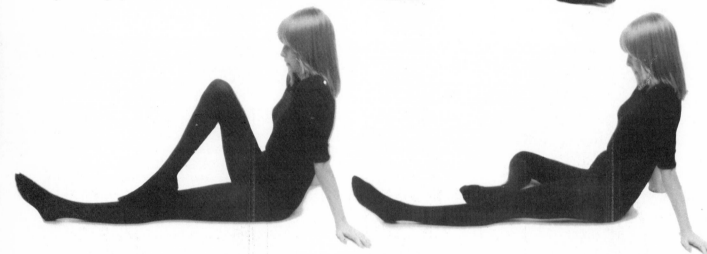

Toe push Lie on the floor on your back with your hands resting under your head. Breathing steadily, move your legs outwards, turning the feet out, too. Now turn your feet so that the insides of the heels press on to the floor. Pushing your heels hard down into the floor, now try to pull your legs together while resisting the movement at the same time. You will feel the muscles of the inner thigh pulling if you are doing this properly. Return to the resting position and repeat five times, gradually progressing to a maximum of 15 times.

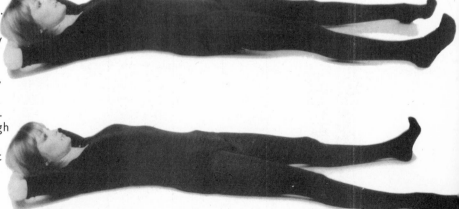

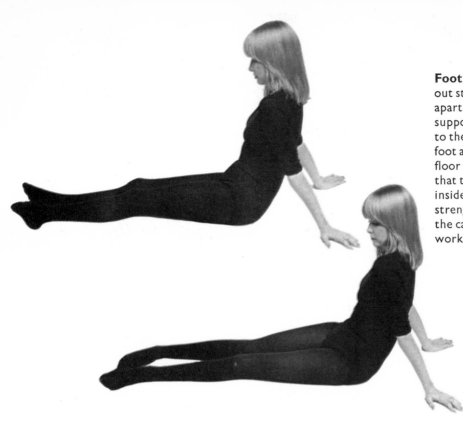

Foot flipping Sit on the floor, with legs out straight and feet about 30 cm [1 ft] apart. Put your hands behind you for support. Breathing steadily, roll the feet to the right so that the outside of the right foot and the inside of the left foot touch the floor together. Roll the feet to the left so that the outside of the left foot and the inside of the right foot touch the floor. The strength should come from the ankles, not the calf muscles. Repeat this five times, working up to 10.

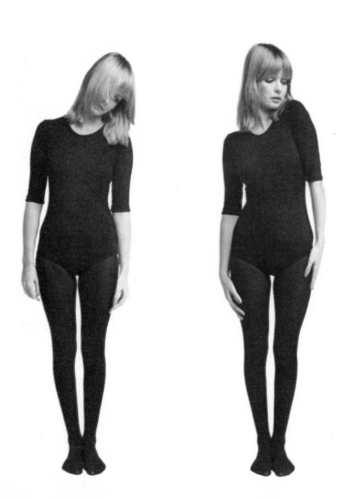

Post work-out relaxercisers
For the neck With a little bounce, drop your head down to the left of your chest. Now drop it to the right of the chest. Raise it again, and do this exercise four times.

For the shoulders Shrug one shoulder at the time, but make it a hard, firm shrug. Do four to six shrugs with each shoulder.

For the breathing Lie on the floor with arms at the sides. Exhale air through the nose. Raise your abdomen as you start to breathe in deeply and slowly, filling your lungs with as much air as you can. Your abdomen should lower as the breathing deepens. Now breathe out slowly. When you have exhaled completely, pull the abdomen in sharply. Gradually relax and repeat the exercise, progressing by one until you are doing it six or seven times.

INDEX